HUMANBIOTECHNOLOGY AS SOCIAL CHALLENGE

Humanbiotechnology has progressed immensely, and humanbiotechnological research has entered a crucial stage. This collection of essays is a significant and original contribution to the public debate on humanbiotechnology and its ethical and social ramifications.

Interdisciplinary in composition this volume brings together leading academics in the fields of biology, law, theology, ethics and sociology to share their viewpoints and insights and to promote exchange between disciplines and convey facts and opinions to the wider public on this increasingly important area of technological development and ethical interest.

Eschewing analysis on pragmatic or utilitarian grounds the essays in this collection are informed by the key ethical concept of 'human dignity' which has been central to the continental debate on human bioethics and is gaining in importance for the debate in the anglophone world.

ASHGATE STUDIES IN APPLIED ETHICS

Scandals in medical research and practice; physicians unsure how to manage new powers to postpone death and reshape life; business people operating in a world with few borders; damage to the environment; concern with animal welfare – all have prompted an international demand for ethical standards which go beyond matters of personal taste and opinion.

The *Ashgate Studies in Applied Ethics* series presents leading international research on the most topical areas of applied and professional ethics. Focusing on professional, business, environmental, medical and bio-ethics, the series draws from many diverse interdisciplinary perspectives including: philosophical, historical, legal, medical, environmental and sociological. Exploring the intersection of theory and practice, books in this series will prove of particular value to researchers, students, and practitioners worldwide.

Series Editors:

Ruth Chadwick, Cardiff Law School, Cardiff University, UK
Dr David Lamb, Honorary Reader in Bioethics, University of Birmingham, UK
Professor Michael Davis, Illinois Institute of Technology, USA

Other titles in the series include:

Liezl van Zyl
Death and Compassion
A Virtue-Based Approach to Euthanasia

Edited by Andreas-Holger Maehle and Johanna Geyer-Kordesch
Historical and Philosophical Perspectives on Biomedical Ethics
From Paternalism to Autonomy?

Stephen Coleman
The Ethics of Artificial Uteruses
Implications for Reproduction and Abortion

Stan van Hooft
Caring About Health

Humanbiotechnology as Social Challenge

An Interdisciplinary Introduction to Bioethics

Edited by

NIKOLAUS KNOEPFFLER
University of Jena, Germany

DAGMAR SCHIPANSKI
Minister of Science, Research, and Art in Thuringia, Germany

STEFAN LORENZ SORGNER
University of Jena, Germany

ASHGATE

Published by
Ashgate Publishing Limited
Gower House
Croft Road
Aldershot
Hampshire GU11 3HR
England

Ashgate Publishing Company
Suite 420
101 Cherry Street
Burlington, VT 05401-4405
USA

Ashgate website: http://www.ashgate.com

British Library Cataloguing in Publication Data
Humanbiotechnology as Social Challenge: An Interdisciplinary Introduction to Bioethics. - (Ashgate Studies in Applied Ethics)
1. Bioethics – Congresses. 2. Biotechnology – Moral and ethical aspects – Congresses.
I.Knoepffler, Nikolaus. II.Schipanski, Dagmar, 1943– . III.Sorgner, Stefan Lorenz.
174.9'57

Library of Congress Cataloging-in-Publication Data
Humanbiotechnology as Social Challenge: An Interdisciplinary Introduction to Bioethics / edited by Nikolaus Knoepffler, Dagmar Schipanski and Stefan Lorenz Sorgner.
p. cm. – (Ashgate Studies in Applied Ethics)
Includes index.
1. Medical ethics. 2. Biology – Social aspects. I. Knoepffler, Nikolaus. II. Schipanski, Dagmar, 1943– . III. Sorgner, Stefan Lorenz.
R724.H795 2007
174'.957–dc22 2006018028

This book has been printed on acid-free paper.

ISBN 978-0-7546-5755-2

Printed and bound in Great Britain by Antony Rowe Ltd, Chippenham, Wiltshire.

Contents

List of Contributors

Anselm, Prof. Dr Reiner, studied Evangelical Theology in Munich, Heidelberg and Zurich before his initial examination in theology in 1990. Afterwards, he became a member of the research team at the Institute for Systematic Theology at the University of Munich under the professorship of Dr Trutz Rendtorff. After receiving his PhD in Autumn 1995, he became Research Assistant at the Institute for Systematic Theology at the University of Munich. In 1998/99 he was granted a deputy professorship in Dresden and another in Augsburg for the following year. Since Summer 2000, he has been Professor for Systematic Theology and Ethics at the University of Jena, and in 2001 he was appointed to the Professorship for Ethics in the Faculty of Theology at the University of Göttingen.

Kähler, Regional Bishop, Prof. Dr Christoph, studied Theology in Jena and Greifswald (1964–69). Afterwards, he carried out research studies in the Faculty of Theology at the University of Jena from 1969 to 1973 and was awarded his PhD in Jena in 1974. He was an assistant at the University of Jena until 1977, before his ordination in October of the same year. He subsequently took over the Rectorship of a congregation in Leipzig. Then, in 1990, he became professor at Leipzig's Ecclesiastical College. In 1992, he was appointed Professor in the Faculty of Theology at the University of Leipzig, and from 1997 to 2000 he served as Deputy Rector responsible for teaching and studies. Currently, he is Bishop of the Evangelical–Lutheran Church in Thuringia.

Knoepffler, Prof. Dr Dr Nikolaus, studied Philosophy and Theology in Würzburg and Rome (1981–90), was Licentiate in Theology (1989) and Philosophy (1990) at the Gregorian University in Rome, and graduated with a degree in philosophy from the Gregorian University in 1992. He was a team member at the Institute for Technology, Theology and Natural Sciences (TTN) from 1996 to 2000 and was appointed Lecturer in Philosophy at the University of Munich in 1998. He then became Deputy Manager at TTN (2000–02) and received an appointment with the Commission for Bioethics with the Bavarian Government in 2001. In 2002, he was a visiting professor at Georgetown University, Washington DC. He was then appointed Professor of Applied Ethics at the Friedrich Schiller University, Jena in that same year and Head of the Ethics Centre. He is also the second Vice President of the German Academy for Transplantation Medicine.

Nida-Rümelin, Prof. Dr Julian, former Minister of Culture, studied Philosophy, Physics, Mathematics and Political Science in Munich and in Tübingen. After graduating and receiving an appointment as a university professor, he was a guest professor in the US and professor at the Centre for Ethics in Science at the University of Tübingen (1991–93). He has held the Chair for Philosophy at Göttingen University since 1993, where he is the successor to Günther Patzig. From 1994 to 1997, he was the President of the Society for Analytical Philosophy. Between 1998 and 2000, he served as Speaker for Culture in Munich. He then served as the German Minister of Culture in 2001–02. He is currently a member both of the European Academy for Sciences and the Arts and of the Brandenburg Academy for Sciences in Berlin.

Nüsslein-Volhard, **Prof. Dr Christiane**, studied in Frankfurt am Main before graduating with a degree in Biochemistry in Tübingen in 1968. In 1973, she received a PhD and continued her research studies in Basel and Freiburg. She was Team Leader at the European Laboratory for Molecular Biology from 1978 until 1981, and also at the Friedrich Miescher Laboratory in Tübingen between 1981 and 1984. She has been the director of the Max Planck Institute for Biological Development, genetics division in Tübingen, Germany since 1985.

She has received many distinctions and awards, including the Leibniz Prize in 1986, the Albert Lasker Award in 1991, and the Nobel Prize for Medicine in 1995.

She is also a member of the Royal Society in England, the National Academy in the US, the *Ordens pour le mérité* in Germany, and the Advisory Committee on Ethics to the German Government.

Romeo Casabona, **Prof. Dr Dr Carlos Maria**, as well as being a doctor of Law and Medicine, is also Professor of Criminal Law at the University of the Basque Region. He is Head of the Inter-University Professorship Foundation BBVA – *Diputación Foral der Bizkaia* (Government of the Basque Province) for Law and the Human Genome at the University of Deusto, Bilbao, Spain and also at the University of the Basque Region. He is Editor of the magazine *Derecho y Genoma Humano* (*Law and the Human Genome*) as well as the series ‘Library for Law and Science’ and ‘Research into Criminal Law’ (published by Comeres, Granada).

In addition, he is a member of the team of consultants in bioethics working on behalf of the Spanish Ministry of Justice; a member of the Committee to the Spanish Government for advice on ethics in the fields of science and technology; and a member of the National Commission on artificial insemination in humans. He is also the former Dean and Director of the Institute of Criminology in the Faculty of Law at the University of Laguna, Tenerife and is a regional court judge in Zaragoza.

Schipanski, **Minister Prof. Dr-Ing. habil. Dagmar**, studied Applied Physics in Magdeburg from 1962 to 1967 and earned her Engineering Diploma in 1967. She carried out further studies at the Institute for Semi-Conductors at the Academy of Sciences in the Soviet Union in Novosibirsk in 1972 and graduated in 1976. She received a professorial appointment in 1985 and was appointed Professor for Solid State Devices in 1990. She was Dean of the TU in Ilmenau between 1990 and 1993, Rector of the TU Ilmenau from 1995 to 1996, and was Thuringian Minister for Science, Research and Art from 1999 to 2004. Since 2004, she has been the President of the Thuringian State Parliament.

She was a member of the Science Council of the Federal Republic of Germany from 1992 to 1998 and was Chairperson from 1996 to 1998. She was also a member of the Berlin–Brandenburg Academy of Science, as well as the UNESCO World

Commission for Ethics in Science and Technology. Since 1998, she has been a member of COMEST, the German Academy of Natural Science Researchers, Leopoldina, in Halle, and has served on the International Advisory Board of the University of the United Nations in Tokyo since 2001.

Beginning in 1999, she has been President of the German National Cancer Institute (*Deutsche Krebshilfe e. V.*), as well as Senator of the Max Planck Society. In 1996, she received the Federal Republic's Cross of Merit, First Class; in 1999, she was awarded the Arthur Burkhardt Prize. Other honours include Woman of the Year and the Prize for European Women – Germany, both awarded in 2000.

Schöler, **Prof. Dr Hans Robert**, received his Diploma in Biology in Heidelberg in 1982; in 1985, he received his PhD, also in Heidelberg. During the following year, he completed a post-doctorate, again in Heidelberg, and in that same year he was appointed Head of the research group at the Boehring Mannheim Research Centre in Tutzing, a position that he held until 1988. Between 1988 and 1991, he was at the Max Planck Institute in Göttingen; from 1991 to 1999, he was Group Leader at the European Laboratory for Molecular Biology in Heidelberg. From 1999 to 2004, he was Professor in the Chair for Reproduction Medicine at the University of Pennsylvania; from 2000 to 2004, he was the Director of the Centre for Animal Transgenesis and Germ Cell Research. Since 2004, he has been Director of the Department of Cell- and Development Biology at the Max Planck Institute for Molecular Biomedicine, Münster, Germany.

Simon, **Prof. Dr Jürgen**, studied Jurisprudence, Economics, Psychology and German Studies in Tübingen, Freiburg and Munich. He passed his first and second state examinations in jurisprudence and received a Diploma in Economics in Munich. He then received his JD (Juris Doctor) from the University of Freiburg. In Hannover, he earned his qualifications to teach at university level in the areas of Civil Rights, Economic Law and IT law in the field of Jurisprudence. He is currently Head of both the Institute for Jurisprudence at the University of Lüneburg and the Research Centre of Bioethics Law, as well as Director of the distance learning programme, 'Conservation Management, Conservation Economy and Conservation Law'. He is also an adviser and counsellor for a large number of authoritative bodies.

In 1998, he received the BAUM Conservation Prize. He has also taken part in a variety of national and international congresses, symposia and workshops in Germany, Europe, Asia and America, and has additionally served as organizer, chairman, director and lecturer at many of these functions. He has also directed a number of research projects for the Office of Technological Assessment in the German Lower House of Parliament, for the Volkswagen Foundation, for the DFG (the German Research Foundation), for the BMBF (the German Ministry for Education and Research), for other Ministries in the German Government, as well as for private companies and academies. He has also worked for the EU Commission and also for various foundations at home and abroad. In recent years, Dr Simon has undertaken research work on rights and ethics in the fields of Biotechnology, the environment, economics and the new information technologies. He is also the author and editor of a number of books and articles in these fields.

Sorgner, Stefan Lorenz, BA, MA, received his Bachelor's Degree in Philosophy from King's College/University of London and his Master's Degree in Philosophy from the University of Durham. He is currently a PhD candidate, lecturer and researcher at the Institute for Applied Ethics at the Friedrich Schiller University in Jena, Germany.

Vattimo, Prof. Dr Gianni, studied Philosophy in Turin with Luigi Pareyson. He carried out research with H.G. Gadamer und K. Loewith in Heidelberg. He has taught at the University of Turin since 1964 and has been Professor for Theoretical Philosophy in Turin since 1982. He was Visiting Professor at several American universities, including Yale University, UCLA, New York University and the State University of New York.

He is the Co-editor of the newspaper *La Stampa* and a member of the scientific advisory board of various journals, including *Der Revista dí estética* and also the *Accademia delle Scienze* in Turin. Other marks of distinction include honorary titles from the University of La Plata in Argentina (1996); Palermo (1998) and Madrid (2003). At present, he is Vice President of the Accademia della Latinità and has been a member of the European Parliament since 1999.

Wanke, Bishop Prof. Dr Joachim, studied Theology at the Philosophical–Theological Institute in Erfurt. In 1966, he was ordained as a priest; in 1969, he was appointed as Assistant and Prefect at the Seminary in Erfurt. In 1980, he received his PhD and qualifications as a university professor and was appointed full Professor for New Testament Exegesis at the Institute in Erfurt. In that same year, he became Ordaining Bishop in Erfurt and in the following year, he was appointed Bishop (1981). He has also been a member of the Studiorem Novi Testamenti Societas (SNTS) since 1978. From 1995 to 2001, he was a member of the Commission on Ecumenical Questions, the Chairman of the Pastoral Commission of the German Conference of Bishops, and the Chairman of the Working Group for Christian Churches (ACK) in Germany.

Winnacker, Professor Dr Ernst-Ludwig, studied Chemistry in Zürich and received his doctorate from the University of California, Berkeley in 1968. From 1968 to 1970, he did a post-doctorate in Berkeley. He was then at the Medical Nobel Institute at the Karolinska Institute in Stockholm from 1970 to 1972. In 1974, he was an assistant at the Institute for Genetics at the University of Cologne, and during that same year he received his credentials to be a university professor. He has been Professor for Biochemistry at the University of Munich since 1980 and Head of the Laboratory for Molecular Biology – Gene Centre at the University of Munich since 1984. He has also been a visiting professor at Harvard Medical School since 1990. On 1 January 1998, he took over as President of the German Research Foundation (DFG) and is also Vice President of the Alexander von Humboldt Foundation.

He was an advisory member of the Enquête Commission in the German Lower House of Parliament on the subject of 'Chances and Risks in Gene Technology' from 1984 until 1987, and was also Vice President of the German Research Foundation (DFG) from 1987 to 1993. Other important positions include: member of the Science and Technology Advisory Board for the Bavarian Minister President; member of the Academy of Natural Science Researchers, Leopoldina; member of the Göttinger and the North Rhine-Westphalian Academy of Sciences. He was awarded the Arthur Burckhardt Prize in April 1994, and has been non-residential Vice President of the Academy of Natural Science Researchers, Leopoldina, in Halle on the Saale since April 1995.

Professor Winnacker is also a member of the following foundations and committees:

Arthur Burckhardt Foundation, Stuttgart – Advisory Board Member
Aventis Foundation, Strasbourg – Trustee of the Karl Winnacker Foundation
Bayer Inc., Leverkusen – Supervisory Board
Advisor for Science and Research to the Bavarian Minister of State for Science, Research and Art
Berlin–Brandenburg Academy, Berlin – full member of the Bioscientific Medical Class
Braunschweig Prize – member of the Jury
Burda Foundation 'Prometheus' – Advisory Board
EleGene PLC, Martinsried near Munich – Supervisory Board
Eppendorf Young Investigator Award, Hamburg – Selection Committee
Evangelical Academy, Tutzing – Trustee
Fondation de la Maison de la Chimie, Paris
German Academy of Natural Science Researchers, Leopoldina, Halle (Saale) – President
Gottlieb Daimler and Karl Benz Foundation, Ladenburg – Trustee
Harvard Medical School – Board of Overseers, Visiting Committee
Herbert Quandt Foundation, Bad Homburg – Advisory Board
Institute of Medicine, National Academy of Science, Washington
Institute of Technology, Theology and Sciences (TTN) – Honourable Chairman
MediGene, Martinsried, near Munich – Advisory Board
Nascacell, Martinsried, near Munich – Scientific Advisory Board
Scientific–Technical Advisory Board to the Bavarian Minister President in Munich

Note to the English Edition

This collection was translated from German into English by Holly Wermter, and we are very grateful to her for such an excellent translation.

In translating the contributions by Nida-Rümelin and Schipanski, her work was supported by that of David McFarland, who was also the main translator of the Schöler article. Vattimo's contribution was originally written by himself in English. However, Holly Wermter revised both the Schöler and the Vattimo articles.

Many thanks to Kerstin May, Gisela Schmidt and René Seidel, who provided substantial assistance with the preparation of the final version of the English edition.

We also wish to thank Paul Coulam from Ashgate Publishing, and Ruth Chadwick, who accepted this collection to be published in her Applied Ethics series, for each of their assistance.

Foreword

> We should not ask the letters of the Latin language how we should speak German, but rather we need to ask our mothers, the children in the street, the ordinary man in the marketplace. We need to watch their lips, see how they speak, and then afterwards translate. Because it is only in this way that they understand and notice that we are speaking German to them.
>
> *Martin Luther, 'Letter about Translating'*

Luther translated the New Testament from Greek into German in Wartburg Castle, thereby making it accessible to a broader public. The Wartburg Conference on Human Biotechnology, which took place from 6 May to 8 May 2004, also wanted to produce a work of translation, this time without regard to the ultimate truth, but rather to critical questions that affect many people today. Prolific scientists presented the results of the most current research, for example stem cell research, in a way that was palatable to the general public. Representatives of the Church and society, lawyers and ethicists also used clear and comprehensible language as they discussed the central issues of this debate and examined whether or not new possibilities offered by human biotechnological research, such as work with stem cells, might be acceptable. We have decided to publish the lectures, making it possible for the general public to take part in this informed reflection, which should serve not to strengthen prejudices, but rather enable society to form an enlightened opinion.

Acknowledgements

We sincerely thank the sponsors of the Wartburg Conference: 'Human Biotechnology as a Social Challenge', whose generous support made this project successful:

- The German Research Society
- The Thuringia Ministry for Science, Research and Art
- The Hertie Foundation
- The Körber Foundation
- The Organizational Platform for Science in Germany
- The Möllgaard Foundation

We are grateful also to the company Lancia for their provision of three first-rate limousines, which contributed to the event's success. Special thanks to Tanja Napiontek, who deserves credit for arranging this.

Many thanks also to Prof. Dr Rolf Gröschner and Prof. Dr Johannes Wöstemeyer, board members of the Ethics Centre at the Friedrich Schiller University in Jena, Germany, who gave us their support during the conference.

We must also thank Dr Stefan Luther, former Director of the office of the Thuringian Ministry for Science, Research and Art, for his tireless support with the conference organization, and Tim Leichter for his hard work on the Wartburg Conference publicity.

A harmonious collaboration on the part of the team in the Department for Applied Ethics at the Friedrich Schiller University also helped to make this project a success. In particular, we would like to thank the following people who were involved before, during and after the conference: Reyk Albrecht, Romy Arnold, Claudia Häfner, Antje Klemm, Kerstin May, David McFarland, Tobias Müller, Markus Peuckert, Robert Ranisch, Gundula Scherf, Gisela Schmidt, Nadja Schmidt, Dr Anne Siegetsleitner and Dr Heiko Ulrich Zude.

The Editors

Acknowledgements

[illegible]

Chapter One

The Wartburg Conference Project: Human Biotechnology as a Social Challenge

Stefan Lorenz Sorgner

The articles in this anthology originate from lectures that were presented during the International Wartburg Conference entitled, 'Human Biotechnology as a Social Challenge'. The conference took place at the hotel in the Wartburg Castle in Eisenach, Germany from 6 to 8 May 2004 and was organized by the Thuringia Ministry for Science, Research and Art, under the direction of its former Minister, Prof. Dr Dagmar Schipanski; the Ethics Centre at the Friedrich Schiller University in Jena, Germany, under the direction of Prof. Dr Dr Nikolaus Knoepffler; the President of the German Research Foundation (DFG), Prof. Dr Ernst-Ludwig Winnacker; and Nobel Prize winner, Prof. Dr Christiane Nüsslein-Volhard.

The choice of the conference's location was significant. The Wartburg Castle is not only located in the geographic heart of Germany, but it also has an important historical tradition. This is the place where Martin Luther translated the New Testament from Greek into German between 1521 and 1522. The Wartburg Conference should also produce a work of translation, albeit a much more modest one. The objective of the conference was twofold. First, we wanted to make the current state of research in the diverse disciplines of human biotechnology understandable and available to an educated public; in this way, public debates can be de-emotionalized. Both intensifying the amount of information conveyed to the public regarding the varying techniques of the diverse fields and opening the door for public discussions about controversial research projects will serve not only to raise the standards of public discourse and make accurate debate possible, but also to facilitate the shaping of political public opinion and aid in the education of the average citizen.

The current president of the German Research Foundation, Prof. Ernst-Ludwig Winnacker, rightly pointed out in his article, 'Beyond the Genome, Beyond the Stem Cell Discussion: Science as a Communication Problem', that often within the ethical discourse pertaining to human biotechnology, 'fantasy, silly gossip, mere utopias, that belong in science-fiction novels',[1] play a large part. He goes on to assert that the current public debate is shaped by 'black-and-white interpretations, absent of grey areas and it does not do justice to the world of complex, genetically influenced

1 E.-L. Winnacker, 'Jenseits des Genoms, jenseits der Stammzelldiskussion – Wissenschaft als Kommunikationsproblem' (Beyond the Genome, Beyond the Stem Cell Debate: Science as a Communication Problem), *ForumTTN* 9 (2002): 40.

phenomena' (Winnacker 2002: 38). The public has been influenced by these hollow arguments. For these reasons, Winnacker contends that this has been largely justified by the fact that the fundamental knowledge relevant to the discussion has not yet been widely disseminated. Many oppose all forms of stem cell research without even knowing what stem cells are, where they can be found, what kinds of stem cells exist, and what possibilities stem cell research could yield. He correctly points out that this ignorance not only makes it possible for irrational blanket arguments to be effective and for meaningless debates to circulate, but is also the reason for a 'deep-seated anxiety, uncertainty, and uneasiness' that 'exists in all segments of the population' (Winnacker, 2002: 40). It is driven by the fear of a 'human factory', of a 'Brave New World', or of a policy of controlled human breeding, decided by the few in power. The main goal of the Wartburg Conference and, therefore, of the corresponding lectures included in this anthology was and is to confront the root of this fear and anxiety; in this way, superficial knowledge will be replaced with genuine knowledge.

Human dignity is one of the central issues of the debate. It not only makes up the groundwork of the German Constitution and the constitutions of many other countries, but also has a prominent position in the Charter of the United Nations. For this reason, a clarification of the principle of human dignity with regard to human biotechnological questions present in Germany can provide an adequate foundation upon which an increase in the international standards of discussion is possible. Furthermore, an informed opinion could facilitate a reasonable, international consensus, which would be acceptable for people from varying cultural backgrounds. However, it requires differentiated applications in the diverse human biotechnological contexts.

The articles that follow present an overview of the main points of the various research areas from noteworthy representatives in the fields of law, theology, society, the natural sciences, and theoretic and philosophical ethics, through which the reader may gain comprehensive insight into the fundamental disciplines involved and their interconnections. With regard to human biotechnology, the areas that have developed especially fast in recent years – for example, stem cell research, which includes therapeutic cloning as well as gene technology – are the focal point of this discussion. Prof. Dr Christiane Nüsslein-Volhard, Director of the Genetics Department at the Max Planck Institute for Developmental Biology in Tübingen, Germany and Prof. Dr Hans R. Schöler, Director of the Cell and Developmental Biology Department at the Max Planck Institute in Münster, Germany, whose experiments with stem cells from mice received international attention, will be presenting the most recent and 'state-of-the-art' research in the natural sciences. In addition to this, the various legal points of view will be presented and discussed. Prof. Dr Dr Carlos María Romeo Casabona, one of the most respected lawyers in the world, will address the international legal state of affairs with regard to human biotechnology. Prof. Dr Jürgen Simon, one of the leading experts in German gene technology laws, will discuss the current legal situation in Germany. The positions of the two major churches in Germany will be represented in a multi-faceted style by the Vice Chairman of the Council of the Protestant Church and State Bishop of Thuringia, Prof. Dr Christoph Kähler, and the Bishop of the Erfurt Diocese, Prof. Dr Joachim Wanke. Insights into the ethical debate will be imparted by the leading theological and philosophical ethicists, including Prof. Dr Reiner Anselm, the Chairman for Ethics in the Theology Department at the University of Göttingen; Prof. Dr Dr Nikolaus Knoepffler, who holds the only Chair in Applied Ethics in Germany at the Friedrich Schiller University in Jena; Prof. Dr Julian Nida-Rümelin, the Chairman of the Geschwister Scholl Institute for Political Science at the Ludwig Maximilians University in Munich; and Prof. Dr Gianni Vattimo, Professor of Theoretical Philosophy in Turin, Italy and former member of the European Parliament. Issues regarding society's responsibility with regard to human biotechnology and an explanation of what needs to be done in order to contribute constructively to an international consensus in conflict situations will be addressed by Prof. Dr Dagmar Schipanski, the current President of the Thuringia Parliament and long-standing Minister for Science, Research and Art in Thuringia, and by Prof. Dr Ernst-Ludwig Winnacker, the President of the German Research Foundation.

Science

In the article by Nüsslein-Volhard, 'Research on Human Embryos?', a general, scientific overview of the controversial research areas in the current bioethical debate will be presented. She points out that some methods, which are, from a biological perspective, not practicable now or in the near future, are illegal. For this reason, it is her mission to pass on basic biological knowledge, which in some cases is nothing new, but has not yet become a part of our general knowledge. Finally, she explains that the field of human embryonic research can be discussed with the help of three essential themes: '(1) diagnostic procedures in IVF or pre-implantation diagnosis; (2) influencing the genetic make-up of human embryos by selection, gene therapy or cloning; and (3) embryonic stem cells for research and therapy.' She also deals with the separate issues in more detail, for example germ cell therapy, which she considers unrealistic with regard to its practicability. Furthermore, she argues that it is a known fact that at this point in time cloning by means of nuclear transfer is successful as an exception, not the rule. Moreover, an improvement of this method is not foreseeable. However, she describes the work of American researchers as promising, who recently had success in propagating embryonic stem cells which could then develop into particular nerve cells. These nerve cells helped to alleviate the symptoms of Parkinson's disease in rats. Likewise, she believes that 'it is imperative that we contribute to very complicated and risky research, certainly before it has been completely successful', because if therapies using human embryonic stem cells were to be developed, they could not be withheld from patients in Germany or other countries with restrictive laws. Her main concern is to proceed with caution and to ensure that potential contributions to medical research aid in the prevention of suffering and pain, and that they themselves are not hindered by fear of misuse.

Following the general overview from Nüsslein-Volhard, Schöler, in his article 'The Potential of Stem Cells: An Inventory', offers in-depth insight into a specific matter. He asserts that according to current estimates, stem cells could help almost half of the US population, which comprises approximately 128 million people.

When the same ratio is applied to Germany, then it would mean the improvement of 38 million lives. He discusses adult and embryonic stem cells and addresses both their potential and the problems that arise in dealing with them. 'Adult stem sells are undifferentiated cells that are present in otherwise differentiated tissue or organs. They renew themselves throughout their life, producing either identical copies of themselves or differentiating into specialized cells of the respective tissues.' Adult stem cells are also pluripotent and can be found in several places in the body, such as in the 'bone marrow, brain, epidermis, blood, liver, skin, eyes, intestine, pancreas and skeletal muscle'. Additionally, they are supposed to have characteristics that make them suitable for transplantation. It might even be possible 'to activate stem cells to produce more growth factors before the transplantation or to change them genetically so that they build important substances for regenerating the tissue'. Embryonic stem cells (ESC) can be found roughly four to seven days after fertilization. Schöler also asserts that human ESC lines were successfully obtained for the first time in 1998. James Thomson demonstrated that human ESC could be used to produce benign tumours (teratomas) made up of complex tissues when injected into mice. Furthermore, bone, tooth, hair follicle and lung tissue were found; others as well. Schöler goes on to say that the results of Thomson's research prove the pluripotency of ESC, but also point to the possibility that life-threatening tumours (teratocarcinomas) could develop in turn. In addition to that he stresses that therapies using ESC have already yielded positive results in mice and rats. Like Nüsslein-Volhard, he mentions the example of the successful treatment of Parkinson's disease in rats. Spinal cord injuries in mice have also been mended, at least in part. 'Murine ESC were also differentiated into insulin-producing cells that after transplantation were able to produce insulin regulation in diabetics at least some of the time.' Schöler also deals with some facets of the cloning issue. He describes reproductive cloning as '[n]uclear transfer for the creation of viable organisms' and remarks that it faces opposition not only with regard to ethical objections, but also for a number of biological reasons. Experiments with animals should have already made it clear that unforeseeable and not immediately apparent problems are to be expected.

Law

In the article 'Human Biotechnology, Transculturality, Globalization and Symbolic (Criminal) Law', Romeo Casabona points out that it might be wise to aim towards an increased integration of laws on human biotechnology in the criminal code. He maintains that international law, with regard to human biotechnology, has supported a viewpoint that crosses cultural boundaries, which has been helped along by an absence of clear ethical guidelines within existing national laws. He asserts that bioethical law for the most part exists as 'soft law', though with a few exceptions, such as the German Embryo Protection Law. He defines a 'soft law' as a 'law without enforcement and serious legal consequences', and one which in all likelihood masks a number of problems. Romeo Casabona brings three soft laws to light: (1) contradictory values inherent in the national legislation of a number of countries; (2) a 'perspective of globalization' that does not cross cultural boundaries; and (3) shelter in 'symbolic law'. In the case of symbolic law, the effectiveness of prosecution is not as important as moral and social disapproval or the pacification of the general public. He warns, however, of the possibility of cultural imperialism as well as particularism, which could arise with the establishment of a transcultural law in the field of biotechnology that is universally legitimate. Though human rights have reached a high level of recognition in international law, it remains necessary to guarantee that the individual is given an even more significant status than it has presently in many in the worldviews of several non-Western countries. Furthermore, the concept of human rights is not a platonic idea, but is instead subordinate to a continuous development. Romeo Casabona refers to responsibility (Jonas), solidarity, justice (Rawls), equality, tolerance (Kaufmann), impartiality and responsibility for future generations (Romeo Casabona) as the requisite principles of our society. The principle of human dignity has also almost reached the status of a universal principle. However, he also calls attention to the fact that within the context of the bioethical debate, references to the term 'human dignity' are misused as blanket arguments.

Simon expresses his views about so-called 'soft laws', for example with regard to the guidelines of the German Medical Association, in his article, 'Human Biotechnology as a Legal Challenge'. He thinks that many problems could be solved with soft law for several reasons: (1) those affected would be able to exercise greater influence; (2) the possibility of direct interference of legislators would be limited; (3) the rules would be easier to modify. Legislation concerning xenotransplantation (donor-organ transplantation) can serve as a model to show that flexible laws are more suitable than comprehensive, individual regulations. He goes on to assert that more open legislation is possible because the German Constitutional Court has not made a statement relating to the issue of human dignity before the fourteenth day after fertilization. If embryos were to be granted this status, then we also need to investigate whether biotechnical research in any way impinges on human dignity. Weighty considerations must also be made particularly with regard to stem cells that are produced from embryos that were not intended for use in transplantation or 'adoption'. We need to examine which of the use of human embryos with the purpose of finding cures and of protecting human dignity or if 'their dying as such' is more consistent with the principle of human dignity. In particular, the right to life needs to be considered in relation to this. According to Simon, a ban on research using imported stem cells is difficult to justify when we measure it against these constitutional criteria. Furthermore, in the case of pre-implantation diagnosis (PID) it is important to note that a woman should be granted the right to make the final decision concerning whether or not she wishes to have the embryo created for that purpose artificially implanted. Under these circumstances, the woman's right to be well informed must be taken into consideration. In order to justify a ban on PID, an embryo at this stage of development must be granted the protection which the principle of human dignity provides. Moreover, the infringement of rights needs to be of more significance than that of the health and dignity of the mother. In Simon's opinion, this is inappropriate and one can hardly expect the mother 'to allow an examination of the embryo in the mother's womb that could lead to a medically induced abortion'.

The Church

In the article 'Human Biotechnology as a Social Challenge: An Inquiry into an Ethical Opinion-building from a Protestant Perspective', Kähler reflects on how this could be realized. He draws attention to three points that can be explained *ex cathedra*: (1) in his letters to the Corinthians, Paul makes an appeal for continuous self-examination; (2) the teachings of the Protestant Church are not hierarchically structured; and (3) for the most part, the foundation of Christian belief allows room for personal discretion and for acting on one's conscience with regard to ethical questions. Kähler describes the general tendency for Church leaders to lean more towards a restrictive stance with regard to bioethical issues, while academic theologians recommend a more liberal point of view. Every Christian reflection about ethical questions is made on the supposition that human beings are God's creation, from which a clear definition of 'human being' proceeds. Nowadays, a more exact description can be found to the idea of human dignity, which can again be explained by the fact that man was made in God's image (Genesis 1). Kähler continues by saying that human dignity is the result of a relationship bestowed to us by God and not the result of a particular ability intrinsic to human beings. Therefore, man must answer to God. In view of this responsibility, he must cultivate his relationship to God, to himself, to his fellow man, and to all of creation. Kähler offers a catalogue of nine questions that might be valuable for the clarification of ethical questions. The answers to a few of these questions make it clear that he leans towards the position that human dignity and the full protection of life should begin at the moment of fertilization. In particular, he points to the following arguments: (1) the biblical tradition, which, from time immemorial, recognizes the care God bestows on the mother's womb; (2) Ottfried Höffe, who claims that 'the law and morals have always recognized the status and rights of the unborn'; (3) 'according to the civil code, the line of succession has always been determined by the exact moment of possible conception'.

Wanke's article, 'Ethical and Theological Challenges to Human Biotechnology: Observations from the Perspective of Catholic Theology', focuses on reflections on human dignity. Wanke accepts the fact that an embryo and a human being are alive in very different ways and that a child is a person, though not in the same way that an adult is a person. Nevertheless, he stresses the need to apply the term 'person' to human life in its various forms and stages of development. The notion that all human beings are equal follows from an understanding of human dignity that is characteristic of the Christian tradition and of the Enlightenment. Moreover, the principle of human dignity has a more fundamental status, is more deeply rooted, and is of greater moral importance than a purely biological understanding of human life. Furthermore, if one is to take the notion of human dignity seriously, one must then ascribe it to all living human beings. Consequently, Wanke holds the opinion that 'it is fair to maintain that human life begins with the fusion of egg and sperm cell, despite unanswered questions. This does justice to the concepts of potentiality and continuity.' With regard to research in the field of human biotechnology, he concludes that, even in the earliest stages of development, human embryos should be granted the same protection rights as other human beings. Regardless of the fact that such research can open the door to new possibilities in the field of medicine, one must always bear in mind that the sacrifice of human life will not be tolerated. At the least, the faithful are aware of the indisposability of human life. It is also worth noting that, apart from the increase in the quality of life, thanks to advances in science and technology, 'the need to accept suffering, to learn how to live with it and to give it meaning' must also be stable and central aspects of society.

Philosophical and Theological Ethics

Anselm deals with some other attitudes concerning the use of the human dignity argument in the bioethical debate in his article, 'Human Dignity as a Regulatory Principle of Bioethics: A Theological Perspective'. First, he discusses two very different currents, which serve as the hallmarks of the current debate. One of the movements is distinguished by an increased exactness with which ethical problems are described. The other development is such that normative concepts are dealt with in an increasingly reductionist method. Applied ethics represents a bridge between descriptive and normative elements. Furthermore, the excessive use of the term 'human dignity' in the field of bioethics is, with regard to ethical reflection, the result of a desire to take the context into consideration, but also to have the same norm as the starting point. The following problem arises from questions pertaining to how the concept of human dignity should be understood. Anselm asserts that only as an empty formula can it develop an integrating effect. However, a specific reason for human dignity is only useful in response to *some* questions; not everyone will consent to a specific reason. Likewise, this means that the basis for the centrality of the human dignity argument would be destroyed because the term's integrating function would be lost. Reference to human dignity within the field of bioethics solely means that ethics is being thematized. Anselm argues against the establishment of a specific argument, which would allow the term human dignity to continue to be used as a reference point for various ethical theories. He hopes that through investigation it may be possible to ascertain the commonalities shared by diverse arguments for human dignity within a given culture. In this way, the idea of human dignity could be connected with the notion of a 'basic ethical consensus'. He doubts, however, that all pertinent problems could be resolved in this way.

As the title of his article suggests, Knoepffler calls for 'Tolerance and Respect in Bioethical Conflicts'. Using the example of pre-implantation diagnosis (here, the internationally recognized abbreviation 'PGD' will be used), he shows how intensely the German debate is shaped by intolerant assumptions and seeks ways to overcome them. He starts out by explaining why the various ethical assessments of PGD are based on arguments that defy consensus. PGD cannot be seen as morally acceptable if artificial insemination is considered immoral. Furthermore, if the protection of human dignity is granted to 6- to 7-celled human embryos, then PGD can be supported only by those who consider it a form of passive euthanasia, at least structurally. Agreeing to certain PGD-related measures if human embryos are not considered to have dignity and if parents are granted the right to make use of modern technology with regard to their offspring is understandable. In this case, it could even be seen as morally untenable to prohibit parents from taking advantage of the technical possibilities. Additionally, Knoepffler emphasizes that, based on current laws, it is not clear whether not yet implanted, fertilized ova are entitled to human dignity. Nevertheless, PGD is being compared with the Holocaust of the Third Reich. Based on the reasons just mentioned, Knoepffler argues for compromise. To ensure that those who oppose PGD do not have to support it financially, it should not be funded by insurance companies. Likewise, PGD should only be permitted in connection with specified objectives.

Nida-Rümelin clearly turns away from all innate-based models of human dignity in his article, 'Human Biotechnology as an Ethical and Social Challenge'. He maintains that innate-based models contain statements about the nature of human being. Instead, he advocates a 'middle-of-the-road' ethics, which follows the example of Rawls's concept of 'overlapping consensus'. Because he thinks it is wrong that in vitro embryos in the early stages of development are granted human dignity, he raises no fundamental moral objection to the decision by the British Parliament, which allows the practice of therapeutic cloning until the point of time at which the fertilized ovum implants itself in the uterus. However, presently he speaks against a plan that the British model be introduced in Germany. With regard to the question of what should happen after PGD, he suggests we should strive towards a 'balanced legal solution'.

Vattimo addresses the issue of 'Bioethics between *Physis* and *Nomos*'. At the centre of his argument is a radical scepticism about the possibility to understand nature. He explains existing concepts of nature with reference to social conditions and contingent interests. His scepticism also concerns the natural right to freedom, upon which modern democracies are built. Likewise, freedom and all of its various connotations is by definition not a 'truth' that must be recognized by a democratic government. Rather, it should be seen more as a practical instrument of the people, through which the authority of those in power can be kept in check. Irrespective of one's understanding of 'democracy', for Vattimo it is significant to note that our culture is marked by democracy and the absence of deep-seated metaphysics. He takes issue with every plea for truth about the nature of humankind and of the world, because these positions are bound together with the existence of an absolute authority. Therefore, he rejects also the idea of an innate human dignity. Instead, he makes an appeal that public discourse and democratic elections decide what appears to be natural or unnatural to a community that defines itself by history. He also supports such a line of action with regard to problems in the field of human biotechnology. In this sense, he concurs with Aristotle's understanding of virtue, and the way in which it explains the notion that in order to find out whether a person is virtuous, one must ask the community. Like Aristotle, Vattimo supports the idea that both the historical context and the current cultural situation must be considered when inquiring about the criteria for 'naturalness'. Consequently, he is opposed to the difference between 'that which grows' and 'that which is made' as found in Habermas's work.

Society

Schipanski's article, 'On the Responsibility of the Scientist', has its origins in the basic values of Christianity, in which Europe has been politically and culturally rooted for centuries. She states that the principle of human dignity has a particular significance: (1) it represents the core of these values; (2) it is the basis of the German Constitution; (3) it is considered to be absolute and universal, which means it is independent of our individual characteristics, cultural makeup and religious convictions; (4) it is a gift from God to humankind.

Freedom and equality, both cardinal values, have their roots in the concept of human dignity. In particular, freedom requires not only responsibility for oneself, but also for one's fellow man and all of creation. For this reason, it is essential that we not only postulate about human dignity, freedom and the willingness to accept responsibility, but we must also actively 'live' these virtues. Schipanski explains that the basis presented here is the ethical and legal foundation upon which further discourses can take place, particularly those fundamental to a democracy. For example, our democracy survives because of diversity of opinions, debate and a struggle for consensus. However, public discourse requires an acquaintance with the latest scientific findings. For this reason, the scientific community has a duty both to make information about the chances and risks associated with new research and findings available to the public, and to explain it. Schipanski also makes it clear that the risks should not be exaggerated, while at the same time the chances should not be underemphasized. Instead, an open, objective, factual and serious discussion needs to take place. Furthermore, because the field of human biotechnology presents us with the power to actively alter human beings, it must be treated with the highest level of sensibility. It would not be in anyone's best interest to completely bar genetic research and the resulting advances in medicine, because gene technology offers new possibilities for relieving pain and for finding cures. As President of the German Cancer Society, she is well aware of this fact.

In his article 'Society's Responsibility in view of New Possibilities in Human Biotechnology', Winnacker points out the merits of the 'escalation model', which was developed in the mid-1990s by himself and some of his colleagues at the University of Munich. One component of this theory pertains to the set of parameters by which the possibilities afforded by genetic engineering can be measured. In this way, a hierarchy regarding the degree of intervention is created. The principles of the escalation model are as follows. First, human dignity prohibits the instrumentalization of human life for objectives that are not related to the person in question. Accordingly, autonomy is given particular importance. In other words, without permission from the patient, no procedure can be carried out. Second, human dignity always comes before the sovereignty of research in the hierarchy of basic rights. Winnacker remains sceptical about several forms of gene therapy. In particular, he considers therapeutic cloning to be a mistake in light of current findings. He also stresses a that ethical considerations regarding the beginning of life are particularly difficult. Nevertheless, he contends that it is wrong to say that an absolute protection of life, including human dignity, should be enforced with the emergence of the zygote. In his opinion, this occurs at the moment the ovum implants itself in the uterus. He justifies his position with the following considerations. First, individuality is a part of being human. This is present only after the point of time at which it is no longer possible for the zygote to develop into twins; that is, approximately fourteen days after fertilization. Second, apart from sperm and an ovum, the uterus is a fundamental condition for the development of a human embryo.

Conclusion

This overview represents a first look at the current state of the bioethical debate in Germany. There are three main positions: on the one side, there is the opinion that an embryo should be given absolute protection, starting at the moment that the genetic material from the sperm and egg cells is united; on the opposing side, others are calling for unrestricted embryonic stem cell research; and in the middle are those urging for compromise, for example that controversial research should not be supported by health insurance companies or tax-payers' money.

PART I
Science

Chapter Two

Research on Human Embryos?

Christiane Nüsslein-Volhard

Biology, the science of life, is currently the subject of intense discussion. This is because discoveries in the areas of embryology, genetics, and – the culmination – the decoding of the human genome serve not only to increase our knowledge, but, in principle, also to open the door to new possibilities for exerting influence on human life. Moreover, these discoveries arouse speculation and fantasy that if they are put to general use, they will decidedly change our world. Although some medical uses of the new technologies, particularly gene technology, have meanwhile gained wide acceptance, concern about both the effects of the new methods and the unforeseeable consequences, despite good intentions, is widespread. For these reasons, the current debate in Germany concentrates on the handling of in vitro human embryos and the possibilities of gene manipulation. Within Europe, the regulations regarding the handling of human embryos are very different. The restrictive laws in Germany and Ireland, for example, stand in contrast to the liberal laws in countries like Sweden or England. As long as no general consensus in this matter, which concerns everyone, is reached, and no reasonable regulations are established that are binding, at least within Europe, then the debate will continue.

So what is it about? Since 1978, it has been possible for the human ovum, still at a very early stage of development, to be fertilized and kept in a culture before it is implanted in the mother in order to initiate pregnancy. As a result, countless embryos that never find mothers are created. This opens up the possibility of using these early-stage embryos for medical research. Embryonic stem cells, which can be used in cell-replacement therapies for the treatment of a range of serious diseases, can be isolated from these embryos. Furthermore, genetic diseases could be avoided, and maybe even eradicated, through genetic diagnosis on these early-stage embryos. However, in the West, our fundamental belief is that one may not sacrifice a human being as a means to an end for other human beings. This ban on instrumentalization provides the foundation for the term 'human dignity', which is inviolable according to our Constitution. The controversy does not concern the recognition of this moral conviction, which both the supporters and opponents, and, of course, our European neighbours have in common; rather, the question is, at what point is human life a human being? Are these early-stage embryos human beings, who are due the same protection as pre-natal foetuses or human beings who have already been born? Or, do they have a lower moral status, which gradually increases until birth? This opinion corresponds most closely with our intuition and plays a role in questions about contraception and abortion laws; the opinions differ considerably on this point. According to the German Embryo-Protection Law from 1990, an embryo at the moment of the ovum's fertilization is granted the same protection as an embryo after the beginning of the pregnancy, whereas other countries grant the embryo protection at the moment of nidation or when the female organism receives the embryo. In England, the law states that an embryo is granted protection from the fourteenth day, at which point the embryo begins to take shape and the window of opportunity for the development of twins is closed. According to the legal definition, a human being is a person only after birth.

These definitions do indeed touch on the biological processes, but concepts such as 'dignity', 'protection' and 'the right to life' are not biological, but moral traits. For this reason, it is not up to the life sciences to answer these questions; it is the responsibility of our society and politicians. That there are striking differences between nations with very similar cultural backgrounds alone makes it clear that there is not one 'right' answer. However, to ensure legal confidence and give research the necessary autonomy, explicit guidelines are required that may be recognized and respected universally. The legal definitions regarding when protection should begin need to be reasonable, plausible and consistent. On this point, biologists could give us information about the degrees or stages of development and maybe also offer recommendations. It is also a scientist's responsibility to inform us about potential applications for the future and the consequences of research on human embryos, which may facilitate logical weighing of arguments for the protection of life against those regarding the recovery of the critically ill.

The differences in legal terminology in the various European countries have nothing to do with varying attitudes of the scientists in these countries. Rather, they correspond to the degree of trust in scientific counsel and in science itself in each country. Are there reasonable grounds for such mistrust? Is it really only a matter of time until the nightmarish visions of science fiction and of utopian novels become reality? Is it even possible that anything we can dream up might be realized? And, above all, will everything that is within our capabilities be implemented even if it is rejected by society? If this were the case, then caution would certainly be necessary, because many of the outlined scenarios are frightening. Nevertheless, it is not likely that research will progress so fast that it becomes no longer possible to establish reasonable and internationally binding regulations for its use within a sufficient span of time. Already, some procedures are prohibited which are at present impossible and in the future will not be practicable. Therefore, it seems as though the problem has nothing to do with establishing regulations within a reasonable time span; instead, a widespread ignorance of the fundamentals of biology abounds. Several important biological principles, some of which have been long known to scientists, have not yet become a part of our general knowledge. For this reason, it may be useful to recapitulate the basic tenets concerning genes and embryos in a modern light.

In the field of biology, discoveries are not continuous, but tend to come in stages. New techniques provide the catalyst for a rapid growth in progress, until a period of stagnation sets in, during which the previous course cannot be continued. The last 150 years can be divided into three major periods. Each of these lasted about fifty years and is marked by significant discoveries that came in surges and gave research new direction.

In the middle of the nineteenth century, Darwin's theory of evolution and the nearly simultaneous discovery that all organisms are composed of cells gave birth to modern biology. During the second half of the nineteenth century, critical discoveries in the areas of genetics and embryology were made, which reached their pinnacle in 1903 with the German biologist Boveri and the American biologist Sutton's formulation of the chromosome theory of heredity. With that, the foundation was laid regarding the understanding of generational succession. From this point on, embryology and genetics developed into separate disciplines. Genetic research blossomed and in 1953 culminated in the unearthing of the molecular structure of genes. This discovery spurred biologists on a great deal, and within a few years they managed to clarify fundamental problems concerning the functions of genes. The development of genetic engineering made it possible to isolate genes, decode their sequences and predict the structure of their protein products. As a result, advances in all areas of biology, unthinkable without genetic engineering, were made possible. Additionally, a number of very complex processes in cell biology, evolution and neurobiology were understandable on the molecular level. In the past few decades, the genomes of various multi-celled organisms, including human beings, have been decoded.

The analysis of several genes in different model organisms and the possibility of comparing corresponding genes in various animals have led to a number of important conclusions, as follows.

1. There is a high level of affinity between the genes of very different organisms. For example, nearly half of the human genes share distinct similarities with those of yeast, flies or worms, and that is also true of any other pair. On the one hand, this relationship means that the proteins that make up every cell have a common origin. This is perhaps not so astonishing because all multi-celled organisms undoubtedly descended from single-celled life forms, which already possessed the essential building blocks of cells. However, the big surprise, which came about twenty years ago as the result of comparative investigations of the genes of various animals, including human beings, was that superordinate mechanisms, which determine an animal's blueprint, are also very similar, although the animals, such as worms, flies and mice, do not look at all alike. Complex interactions of proteins often play a role with regard to these mechanisms, and what is remarkable is that one finds them in the same or a very similar correlation in distantly related species. With that in mind, corresponding genes in humans, mice and flies are only in very rare instances exactly the same, but the fact that they can be traced to a common origin is still recognizable. This means that during the process of evolution, with the genesis of new species, molecules often preserved their interactions, though they were also modified, doubled, lost or newly combined; only rarely did something completely new occur.
2. Most genes play a role in several and frequently innumerable processes, in various organs and at various times. Furthermore, animals have astoundingly few genes. A fly, for example, has 13,000 and a mouse or a human being has 32,000. What this means is that one gene in an organism typically takes

> on several functions, and the connection between a physical property and a gene is not direct, but rather exists on multiple levels. Thus, modern genetic research confirms the observations of classic genetics. As a rule, each gene has an influence on several physical properties, and, conversely, every physical property is dependent on several genes. What this means for human beings is that there is no single gene for certain characteristics such as nose length, blood sugar level, musicality and so on; rather, both physical and mental traits depend on the constitution of numerous genes. This also indicates that with a single gene, be it from a mouse or a human being, one could probably not predict with accuracy everything it influences.

In 1999, the genome sequence of the first multi-celled organism, the threadworm *Caenorhabditis elegans*, was decoded. Since then, other genomes have been fully analyzed, including those of flies, human beings and mice. This international programme of genome research has given scientists a lot to do in the coming years, because this enormous amount of information needs to be understood in order to be useful.

The human genome is currently the largest to have been decoded. Although it is bigger and more complexly constructed, human genes are not always different from those of animals. It is also clear that an organism's complexity is not really reflected in the number of genes it has. For example, a simple worm has 19,000 genes, and a human being, with 32,000, does not even have twice as many. With the help of the gene sequence alone, the biochemical properties of the protein product can be derived, at most. That is clearly insufficient for making assumptions about the consequences of a gene modification or breakdown in a human being, and conversely it means that the gene analysis of a single person hardly allows one to make predictions about his or her makeup. At present, it is impossible to say how our ignorance with regard to the exact functions of human genes will change in the future. Research that experimentally or genetically intervenes in the life of organisms with calculated and necessary control should be prohibited for use on human beings. From a biological standpoint, human beings are vertebrates like frogs, chickens and fish, and much can be learned about both vertebrate-specific processes and human biology through research on these animals.

Animals are composed of cells that divide and develop from simple to more complex forms in the course of embryonic genesis. An individual begins his life as a fertilized ovum; a form that is in no way similar to the structure and shape of the animal that will eventually develop. A cell is the smallest unit of an organism, and every cell has an outer membrane and a nucleus and is filled with cytoplasm. The nucleus contains thread-shaped structures, called chromosomes, which are not visible in a latent cell. In the middle of the nineteenth century, topics such as whether cells could renew themselves and whether chromosomes survive or dissolve after cell division were still being debated. At some point in the middle of the nineteenth century, it was shown that every cell originates as a result of this cell division process (*ominis cellula e cellula*) and that cells and organisms cannot evolve from dead material in a process of abiogenesis (spontaneous generation). During cell division, the chromosomes first double lengthwise, and then a copy is passed on to both daughter cells. This mechanism ensures that the daughter cells receive the same chromosomal make-up as the mother cell. Furthermore, because chromosomes are the carriers of the genes, this means that the daughter cells, which developed as a result of the division of the mother cell, have the same repository of genes as the mother cell.

The development of an animal begins with the fertilization process, which is the fusion of egg cell and sperm. This produces a zygote, whose cytoplasm comes from the ovum, but whose nucleus consists of an equal amount of maternal and paternal chromosomes. The fertilized egg cell divides several times, and at the beginning of the process all of the cells look identical. After a short time, however, the cells start to differentiate themselves and the embryo begins to take shape. The cells separate into groups; synthesize with or fold themselves into the embryo; push against each other; continue dividing; and form organ and tissue structures. Eventually, the cells differentiate themselves, so that they can fulfil their various functions within the animal.

The realization that every cell has all the chromosomes and thereby all the genes of that organism, despite the fact that the cells develop in diverse ways and can look very different, was very important. An organism is composed of a large number of hereditarily identical cells and is, therefore, a clone, which springs from a parent cell, the fertilized ovum. The British scientist John Gurdon tested this theory. Using frogs, he transplanted skin cell nuclei or larvae into egg cells whose nuclei had been deactivated. In rare cases, these cells developed into a frog. With this, he showed that, in principle, the various cells contain all the genes. The resulting frog is hereditarily identical to the donor of the skin cell; in other words, it is its clone. Recently, even cloned mammals managed to reach adulthood (the famous sheep, Dolly), but again the success rate was extremely low and to this day has not substantially improved. The problem is not that the method is not well tried, but that in nature reproduction does not occur through cloning; it is the result of sexual reproduction. This is because particular cells are separated from the body's cells for reproductive purposes. These 'initial germ cells' migrate to the sex organs, where they will later form ova and sperm. This germ line and the somatic cells are called soma. Because offspring develop out of the germ cells, gene mutations are inherited only when they turn up in the germ line cells. Therefore, acquired characteristics cannot be inherited! The germ line goes through a special developmental programme, in which its genome is protected so the cells that create the next generation remain as intact as possible. Somatic cells are not protected from mutations in the same way, and, depending on age, they contain a number of mutations, which are not detrimental to the individual cells, but only in rare cases can guarantee the normal development of an animal. This explains cloning's extremely low success rate, which defies improvement.

At various stages of its life, an animal can look very different although it has the same genes – for example, a caterpillar and a butterfly or a maggot and a fly. If every cell contains every gene, one must take a look at the cytoplasm for the cause of this cell differentiation during development. Factors in the cytoplasm determine what the cell will become and ultimately which genes will be expressed. The daughter cells, which develop when a frog ovum divides for the first time, could also develop into an entire, albeit smaller, frog. However, this is no longer possible after a few divisions.

Boveri observed that an egg has polarity and that an artificial division across the axes cannot result in a fully fledged embryo. Afterwards, the right side and above and below the axes are already different. Cytoplasmic factors, which gradually increase or decrease from top to bottom, determine the developmental fate of the cells they surround in various ways. The secret of development is the ability to control the genes in time and space. Together with cytoplasmic factors, which control the genes, the genes function as blueprint for the developing organism, which comes into being as the result of consecutive stages, each building on the one before. A cell is also stimulated, or rather it receives signals, from outside and from neighbouring cells, which are passed on to the genes in the nucleus. This means that the fate of a cell is not only dependent on cytoplasmic factors, but also on external circumstances. The nucleus, as well as the genes, contains all of the hereditary information for the developmental programme.

Experiments that study embryology and development, such as those performed on animals, are banned for use on human beings. As we have seen, however, many of the fundamental mechanisms of development are shared by differing species, and for this reason we can learn a lot from experiments on vertebrates, such as frogs, chickens and fish. Without a doubt, the very early development of mammals, including human beings, is special, and mice are the best model organisms.

What is so special about the development of mammals? Frogs, birds and fish lay eggs shortly after fertilization, which contain both the genetic programme and all of the nutrients and factors necessary for the development of a self-sufficient chick or tadpole outside the mother. The deposited egg's external needs are little more than a particular temperature, moisture and air in order to nurture an independent being. This is not true of mammals because mammals are viviparous, which means that from fertilization until birth the embryo develops and is nourished inside the mother's womb. The development takes places in two phases. In the first phase after fertilization, the ovum's cytoplasm contains only the information needed to form a blastocyst, made up of little more than 100 cells. At the beginning of the second phase, the actual embryonic genesis, the blastocyst nests itself into the mother's uterus. Nourished by the mother's womb, where the embryo develops, it takes shape and grows. Consequently, in mammals there is a characteristic delay in the care of the embryo by the mother, which is relative to the moment of fertilization. The process of equipping the egg with nutrients for the forthcoming embryo, which for egg-laying animals takes place before fertilization, in mammals is postponed until after the fertilized ovum is implanted in the uterus.

Compared to other animals, the ova of mammals are tiny, and their cytoplasm contains no more information than that needed for the formation of a blastocyst, when the embryo is composed of roughly 100 cells. This comprises only two different cell types. The outer cells will eventually develop into parts of the placenta, which is a structure that is not part of the embryo, but works together with the female organism to facilitate the embryo's nourishment. The inner cells later become the embryo as well as to various protective membranes. The early development into a blastocyst can also take place in vitro, and in many respects it distinguishes itself from that of other vertebrates, in which no difference is made between inner and outer cells and no placenta forms. The fate of the first cells produced during divisions in the zygote is not yet sealed; rather, they remain pluripotent during the course of several cell divisions. In mice, for example, the amalgamation of two genetically different marked embryos in the eight-cell stage can show that the cells are still capable of developing into every structure of the animal, including the germ cells. During this phase, the removal of one or two cells does not harm the embryo because the remaining cells are able to form an entirely normal body. Even the fate of the blastocyst's inner cells is not yet sealed, and their offspring can contribute to every structure, including germ line cells or an embryo's protective membranes.

In order to continue the development process, the blastocyst is implanted in the uterus, where it is nourished from the mother. Additionally, the blastocyst slips out of its shell and penetrates the uterine wall with its outer cells. The embryo develops in close contact with the uterine wall tissue, which stimulates its growth, and both the outer cells and the uterine wall tissues eventually form the placenta. The uterus, supported by the mother's circulatory system, protects and nourishes the growing embryo. The supply of oxygen and nutrients, as well as the removal of metabolic products, takes place through the blood vessels. In this way, the embryo uses the mother's organs – such as the lungs, liver and kidneys – until its own organs are functional. After the fertilized ovum has been implanted in the uterus, several cell layers that enclose the embryo and connect themselves to the placenta evolve from the internal cell mass. Only a small number will eventually form a cell layer, called the epiblast, which corresponds to the gastrula of other vertebrates, out of which the various embryonic structures develop. At this point, the amnion, which is a skin that eventually envelops the embryo, forms above the epiblast. Very early in the development, somewhere around the fifth week after fertilization in human beings, fundamental form-building has taken place, although the embryo is still minute, no more than a few millimetres long. Further development consists of the growth and final differentiation of the embryonic structures.

There are no experiments on human beings that can offer information about the developmental potential of cells during the early stages of embryo development. However, observations of twins allow for interesting inferences. Identical twins are genetically alike, and therefore are produced by the fission of the ovum's offspring. The latest point at which twins can still form (though only in rare cases) is after the formation of the amnion, which occurs after implantation in the uterus, about fourteen days after fertilization. What this means is that even at such a late stage there is still no individual embryo and that the cells of the epiblast have not yet succumbed to their future fate. As already mentioned, according to British law, this is the point at which the protection of life begins.

Research on Human Embryos?

In this section, I shall address the main domains of application in dealing with human embryos that are based on methods compiled from animal models. The procedure of fertilizing human ova in vitro and cultivating them until implantation was developed in England. Then, in 1990, a law was passed there, allowing research on embryos as long as it served to improve in vitro procedures leading in the direction of a cure for infertility, with the understandable reasoning that patients should only be offered therapies that have been researched and tested. In Germany, the Embryo Protection Law from the same year bans any research on embryos, but artificial fertilization (in vitro fertilization, IVF) is permitted and frequently used.

In essence, three main themes are discussed with regard to dealing with human embryos:

(1) diagnostic procedures in IVF or pre-implantation diagnostics;
(2) influencing the genetic make-up of human embryos by selection, gene therapy or cloning; and
(3) embryonic stem cells for research and therapy.

Pre-Implantation Diagnostics

The goal of research (outside Germany) is to increase the rate of successful pregnancies through in vitro fertilization. What this means is that the conditions of the cell culture and the implantation procedures using cultures from the uterine wall are being investigated. This is know in the press as an 'artificial uterus', but it is far from that. Diagnostic procedures were developed in order to identify embryos with certain genetic defects; in pre-implantation diagnostics (PID), a cell is removed when the embryo is at the eight-cell stage, so a genetic test can be performed. As already mentioned, the embryo is not harmed during this procedure. Two indicators are of particular importance in PID:

(1) In human ova, the number of chromosomes often deviates from the norm, due to unavoidable errors in chromosome separation during the ovum's maturation. Because such embryos have no chance of survival, this is a key reason for the low success rate even in normal pregnancies, though in particular among older women. The ability to diagnose damage to chromosomes in advance could increase the number of successful pregnancies. With the help of PID, the frequency of highly problematic multiple births, which occur because more than one embryo is usually implanted with the hope that at least one will develop, can be reduced.
(2) In rare cases in which both partners are carriers of the same serious congenital disease, the embryo has a one in four chance of acquiring the disease according to Mendelian Laws. This can be diagnosed, and only healthy embryos (with regard to the disease in question) are implanted. This type of PID is banned in countries with strict laws, such as Germany. However, foetuses with congenital diseases can be identified during the pregnancy through pre-natal diagnosis and are typically aborted. An early diagnosis before implantation could prevent the killing of such foetuses already at an advanced stage of development.

Influencing the Genetic Make-up of Human Embryos

Selection Misgivings about the introduction of PID are chiefly grounded in fear of misuse; more specifically, that the scope of application could be expanded to include mild defects and that gene constellations other than those found in the mutations of congenital diseases will be selected for experimentation. In a 'designer baby' utopia, we are playing with other types of genes; not with those that lead to disease when defective, but rather with genes that determine a person's healthy traits. We understand these genes the least, and there is little chance to identify them. Experiments on animals do not offer much help, because mice do not have any of the traits that interest us. Consequently, it is not easy to know which individual traits a human being will possess, and even if the DNA is analyzed we cannot know for certain how a human being might turn out if a few of his genes were to exist in alternate forms.

It is at this point that the narrow natural limitations set the bounds of our visions:

- One cannot select a genetic variation in an embryo that is not present in the parents.
- A diagnosis can only be made on a gene, not a trait, and the relationship between genes and traits is very complex.
- Many traits come about through a constellation of several genes, which are typically found in different chromosomes and are distributed in the germ cells independent of each other. Based on purely statistical grounds, the desired constellations are decidedly rare.
- Even when genes completely correspond, as in the case of identical twins, knowledge of the traits of one does not allow for predictions about the traits of the other. What this means is that several non-genetic factors are important and that, on the basis of the gene constellation, many traits are, in principle, unpredictable.

Gene therapy in the germ line For similar reasons, the thought of genetic manipulation in human beings through genetic selection is relegated to the realm of science fiction. It is impossible to guarantee the success of such a process; additionally, it is a weighty factor to consider that up until now there has been no procedure that has enabled the copy of a gene to be introduced in an organism, so that all the cells receive the gene and no unpleasant side effects occur. This requires an explanation: it is certainly possible to infiltrate genes in mice, flies and fish, so why not in humans? The reason is that an accurate genetic transfer occurs very rarely, and success can be measured only in the offspring of the initially treated animal. This means that experiments with animals take place over several generations, and success is accompanied by a large number of unsuccessful attempts. In experiments with human beings, the demands for security and success rates are completely different from those with regard to attempts on animals. It is impossible to 'treat' a particular ovum with still unknown traits and genetic make-up with a success rate of 100 per cent. What this means is that what is 'acceptable' for animals is completely unfeasible for human beings. Furthermore, if the parents are healthy, then there are also healthy embryos which can be selected after diagnosis, thereby making a risky therapy unnecessary.

Somatic gene therapy In principle, it is possible or at least imaginable that a cure for some genetically contingent diseases could be found, in which cells that carry the normal gene are introduced into the patient, and if a portion of the cells are normal they secrete a product that can 'heal' the other cells. Since the isolation of the first defective genes, there has been intensive work on the development of such procedures. However, these have been successful only in rare instances, although there are no ethical objections. Up to this point, the procedures have also been risky because the construction of the gene within the cells is not always perfect and some cells later develop into tumours. Somatic gene therapy is one example of the difficulty in anticipating the success of a direction of research. When research began twenty years ago, it looked as though it would lead to efficient and effective therapies within a few years. Recent reports should have a sobering influence on modern research's often overly optimistic promises for cures.

Cloning In humans, cloning would result in the creation of a human who is genetically identical to an already existing one; in other words, a belated twin. During this process, an embryo would be produced through the transfer of a nucleus from somatic cells into an enucleated ovum. And as I have already mentioned, only in very rare cases does the cloning of animals result in healthy 'offspring'; most of the attempts end in miscarriage or deformity. In the case of Dolly, more than 200 ova were treated, and in most cases the embryo terminated its own development sooner or later or resulted in a deformed animal. There are several reasons for this. One has already been discussed, namely the possibility that mutations had accumulated in the somatic cells whose nuclei had been removed, which in turn interfered with the viability of the embryos produced during the nucleus transfer. Another reason is that somatic cells are already restricted with regard to their development potential. Their genes are wrapped up with specific proteins and are to some extent modified. This restriction must be completely reversed on contact with the ovum's cytoplasm, and this seems to occur only in rare instances. A third reason for the lack of success is that after the transfer of the nucleus into an enucleated ovum, an accurate chromosome division only rarely transpires in the daughter cells. In any case, it is clear that up to this point the success of cloning through nucleus transfer is the exception, not the rule, and it is not foreseeable whether and how the procedure can be improved. Although it is essentially futile to rack our brains over ethical objections to a non-applicable procedure that will never become widespread, the human imagination has been so stirred up that countless ethical debates over cloning have taken place and will continue to do so. Apart from the low success rate and anticipated damages, from the standpoint of biology the greatest concern is the parentless children that would be produced. And the reasons that would prompt someone to duplicate his or herself or another being do not bode well for the well-being of the child. On ethical grounds, human cloning is rejected by researchers worldwide and is strictly banned in many countries, including those with more liberal legislation.

At the centre of the debate is so-called therapeutic cloning in which only a blastocyst is produced by means of nucleus transfer, which then serves medical purposes. A nucleus would be removed from the patient's somatic cells. The goal of this procedure is to generate an embryonic stem cell culture from the blastocyst. (I shall address this later in more detail.) It is likely that the immune system would not reject such stem cells, which would otherwise hinder these kinds of cell therapies. Recently, researchers in Korea managed to produce blastocysts using the method of nucleus transfer, though still with a low success rate.

These kinds of attempts are banned in countries with restrictive legislation, because, *per definitionem*, a human being would be produced and shortly thereafter destroyed. However, this type of research is permitted in England and Sweden, because according to the laws in these countries a blastocyst is not yet granted the protection of an embryo; instead, it is seen as a group of cloned cells from the donor.

Embryonic Stem Cells

A blastocyst's inner cells can be propagated in the culture medium of a Petri dish without changing their embryonic and undifferentiated status. These are the embryonic stem cells or ES cells that have been produced in mice for the last twenty years. When these cells are transplanted into the blastocyst of a host embryo, they begin to develop exactly like the cells of the host. This means that they are pluripotent; in other words, they are still very adaptable. Embryonic stem cells have special traits that present unique research possibilities, because they multiply freely in a culture without changing these traits. When particular factors are added, the development of certain cell types is stimulated while the development of others is suppressed. These experiments have tremendous significance not only for basic research, but also for the evolution of therapies dependent on cell replacement.

A very significant property of embryonic stem cells is that foreign genes are able to infiltrate their genome. This is achieved by the introduction of DNA produced in vitro. In rare cases, the foreign DNA integrates itself in the correct position within the genome, in a process called homologous recombination. These cells can be identified and singled out from the frequent failed attempts. Then the cells are able to grow in a medium in which only the cells that correctly integrated the new gene divide and reproduce. These cells can be transplanted into a blastocyst and can develop into a mouse. A portion of the cells from this chimera derives from the genetically altered cells. When the germ cells are among these cells, the genetically altered status will be securely passed on to the offspring. Presently, this procedure has vast relevance with regard to the analysis of the function of genes, which, except for their DNA sequence, remains largely unknown. It is plausible that in the future the possibility to generate genetic changes in ES cells will play a greater role in the use of these cells in cell therapies for human beings.

Human ES cell cultures have existed since 1998, but because they are not easy to produce and because of countless ethical reservations, research on them has not progressed very far. Diseases in which specific cell types degenerate and are not replaced by the body, such as childhood diabetes, Parkinson's disease and multiple sclerosis, represent the primary fields of application. These are diseases for which there is still no cure. American scientists recently succeeded in reproducing stem cells and were able to differentiate them to specific nerve cells in a cell culture. This significantly reduced Parkinson's disease symptoms in laboratory rats. Current attempts with Type 1 Diabetes are equally promising.

There are also other types of stem cells in other tissues, the so-called adult or somatic stem cells. These typically multiply by means of asymmetrical cell division, in which one daughter cell survives as a stem cell, while the other, usually after several divisions, develops into a differentiated cell, which has the function of replacing dying cells in the tissue. In contrast to ES cells, somatic cells are limited in their developmental potential. Additionally, it is not easy to reproduce them in a culture without changing their properties and it is also difficult to steer them into a different developmental direction. Although research on adult stem cells is generously supported, results comparable to research on ES cells have not yet been achieved. Therefore, it is likely that the first effective therapies for a number of acute diseases will be developed using ES cells, or in any case before therapies with adult stem cells are developed.

Creating human embryonic stem cell cultures is banned in Germany, and a new, very strict law regulates research on imported cultures, which need to have been produced before 1 January 2002. These laws represent an unreasonable compromise, which is clearly reflected in politicians' mistrust of researchers. Consequently, these rules prevent German scientists from keeping up with international research in this field. Nonetheless, it is clear that therapies based on human ES cells, whether developed in England, Sweden or Korea, cannot be withheld from German patients or patients from other countries with restrictive laws. In light of this, it is imperative that we contribute to very complicated and risky research, certainly before it is completely successful. It is at the very least morally questionable for us to profit from research in other countries when it is banned in our country, as in the case of in vitro fertilization.

The Moral Status of Embryos

As already mentioned, with regard to all the legal discrepancies, the main question concerns an embryo's moral status. At what point does a human being have the right to life and the protection of its dignity? As already discussed, it is not the biologists' job to answer this question and the differences in assessments resulting from varied legal terminology does not in any way correspond to the diverse, nationally governed opinions of the scientists. However, it is noteworthy that the pertinent arguments from moralists and philosophers fall back on biological explanations, which do not stand up to scrutiny. A common ethical dogma establishes the point at which an embryo should be protected, with the assertion that, starting from fertilization, human development is a continuous process, without any abrupt turning points or additions that would justify a change in status. It is also argued that the potential for becoming human is completely present with the formation of the zygote and thus with the creation of the developing organism's genome; at this stage, everything which determines a human being is in place. It is quite clear that, after fertilization, a chicken egg has the potential to develop continuously until the chick hatches without the help of the mother, because the egg, equipped with all the necessary nutrients, has already left the mother. In human beings (and other mammals), the embryo, after a short developmental phase in the ovum, must nest itself in the mother in order to continue developing until birth. A zygote has the potential only to develop into a blastocyst, which has to hatch out of the egg casing in order to begin the next stage of development, commencing with nidation. From a biological point of view, there is nothing discontinuous in a developmental process in which an embryo repositions itself into direct cellular contact with another organism. The complete genetic programme is already present in a fertilized ovum. To reach its potential, the embryo needs intense interaction – that is, symbiosis – with another organism, which is the mother in this case. This symbiosis is inimitable and indispensable, and consequently the developmental programme is complete only at the time of the nidation; at birth, the programme is realized. The developing human being is only after the birth a separate, self-sufficient organism that breathes and has its own metabolism. Of course, the infant still has needs, but it receives nourishment from without and can live without its mother in emergency situations. No later than then is a human being a person with full rights, and on that point we are certainly all in agreement.

It is worth noting that the assessment of an embryo's right to protection is in other countries very different from in Germany. The tenor of liberal abortion laws and restrictive embryo-protection laws is extremely varied. The current laws always lead back to strange contradictions, inconsistencies and double standards that likely originate in the inclination to mediate between the two extreme positions. Nevertheless, one can hope that at least in Europe there will soon be valid and plausible regulations, based on conceivable, reasonable and well-thought-out principles. On the one hand, these rules must serve to prevent misuse, but on the other hand, they must not also hinder medical research, which according to ethical imperatives is orientated towards healing. In addition to proving the scientific quality of the intended research, such rules should require that the permission to work with in vitro human embryos is dependent on ample experience with corresponding animal experiments, which promise an acceptable success rate. Such laws must also include rules that forbid the implantation of embryos in a female organism in order to induce pregnancy when something was added to the embryo in vitro, such as chimeras that are diffused with ES cells or were produced by the process of nucleus transfer. Such regulations would include de facto a ban on cloning through both nucleus transfer and ES cells. However, pre-implantation diagnosis would be permitted because the embryo is not harmed by the removal of cells. The main concern is to proceed with caution; to ensure that the potential contributions to medical research prevent pain and suffering, and are not prevented themselves due to fear of misuse.

Chapter Three

The Potential of Stem Cells: An Inventory

Hans R. Schöler

Practically unknown to the public until a few years ago, 'stem cells' have become a magic formula that is expected to solve nearly all of our medical problems in the future.[1] According to current estimates, in the US more than 128 million people could be helped through stem cells. That is about half of the population. Based on this percentage, in Germany that would mean more than 38 million people. The following review of stem cell research presents what is possible, or at least what is within the realm of possibility, and where the limits of the impossible lie (Kirschstein & Skirboll 2001). This paper also provides a basis for ethical and socio-political discussion, although that is not the subject of this scientific review per se.

Adult Stem Cells

The hope that many illnesses may one day be treated with stem cells is based essentially on years of success with bone marrow transplants. More than forty years ago, it was determined that blood-forming stem cells, called haematopoietic stem cells, are responsible for the success of bone marrow transplants in transplanted material (Till & McCulloch 1961: 213–22). The field of stem cell research experienced an enormous boom about four years ago when publications suggested that adult stem cells could differentiate into several different cell types. Until then, this capacity had appeared to be restricted to embryonic stem cells.

Adult stem cells are undifferentiated cells that are present in an otherwise differentiated tissue or organ. They renew themselves throughout their life, producing either identical copies of themselves or differentiating into specialized cells of the respective tissues (Watt & Hogan 2000: 1427–30). Adult stem cells have been discovered in a variety of organs and tissues: bone marrow, brain, epidermis, blood, liver, skin, eyes, intestine, pancreas and skeletal muscle. The use of adult stem cells

1 This paper is based on a lecture given upon the 122nd meeting of the Society of German Biological Researchers and Physicians (GDNÄ) in *Halle*, Germany. It was published in the collection, 'An den Fronten der Forschung – Kosmos-Erde-Leben' ('On the Frontiers of Research: Cosmos-Earth-Life') (S. Hirzel Verlag, Stuttgart, Leipzig, 2003) and in *Naturwissenschaftlichen Rundschau* (*Natural Sciences Review*) 56 (2003): 525. We would like to thank the Journal *Bundesgesundheitsblatt, Gesundheitsforschung, Gesundheitsschutz* for making this article available for publication, 47:6 (2004): 565–77. Copyright Springer-Verlag, 2004.

as therapy for human diseases would be of interest for several reasons. One reason is that it is the function of adult stem cells to build different cell types of a particular tissue. Ideally, it should then be possible through the transplantation of adult stem cells to regenerate all these different cell types. Among other findings, it has been shown that at least a few stem cells can migrate to impaired tissues (Aboody et al. 2000: 12846–51). This would ease surgery significantly because the transplanted tissues would need to match the target tissue less precisely. In addition, it was proven (at least for neural stem cells) that stem cells secrete growth factors that possibly protect or even mobilize other cells in affected tissues (Noble 2000a: 369–70, and 2000b: 12393–5). Should this discovery prove generally valid, the healing of affected tissues could be made easier through this method. It may even be possible to activate stem cells to produce more growth factors before the transplantation or to change them genetically so that they build important substances for regenerating the tissue.

Box 1:

The Term 'Potency' in Developmental and Cell Biology

'Potency' in developmental biology refers to the ability of particular cells and tissues to differentiate. In some organisms, cells undergo an ever-stronger narrowing of their developmental possibilities with each cell division. A well-known example is the firmly determined development of thread worms, in which the cell's 'fate' is determined quite early. In other organisms, such as vertebrates, cells maintain a certain degree of freedom so that they retain the ability, depending upon the development stage (though sometimes lifelong) to replace other cells. This ability contributes, for example, to the high regenerative capabilities of amphibians. This ability to differentiate decreases from totipotent (or omnipotent) to pluripotent, multipotent, oligopotent and unipotent, though the boundaries are not always clear and depend on many external factors (the conditions of the culture, preparation, and so on).

Totipotence (Omnipotence): (a) the ability of a single cell to construct a complete, viable organism, such as a fertilized egg cell; (b) the ability of a stem cell to differentiate into every cell type of an organism. Embryonic stem cells in vitro are a possible example. However, it is experimentally difficult to prove that a cell can in fact differentiate into every different cell type of an organism. Until this is proved, we call this pluripotency.

Pluripotence: the ability of a cell to differentiate into nearly all cells, for example the descendants of each of the three blastodermic layers. This phenomenon can be seen in embryonic stem cells, among others.

Multipotence: the ability of a cell to differentiate into a number of descendents, for example the stem cells of the haematopoietic system (see Fig. 1).

Oligopotence: the ability of a cell to differentiate into a few descendents, for example lymphoid or myeloid stem cells (see Fig. 1).

Unipotence: the ability of a cell to form its own type of cell, for example fibroblasts.

It was astounding that even adult stem cells in a fully grown organism still have a high level of plasticity. Plasticity is the ability of a cell to develop not only into cells of the tissue type in which the cell is found, but also into cells of other tissues. Depending on the degree of plasticity, the cells are referred to as unipotent, oligopotent, multipotent or pluripotent (see Box 1; Boiani & Schöler 2002). The fact that adult stem cells possess pluripotence was surprising and nearly unimaginable; of course, it had also been assumed that stem cells descending from one of the embryo's three germ layers (ectoderm, mesoderm or endoderm) could not generate offspring of one of the other two germ layers. Several researchers have refuted this assumption. Stem cells from bone marrow, which originate in the mesoderm, can differentiate into primary cell types of the brain (neurons, glia cells and astrocytes), all of which originate in the ectoderm (Mezey et al. 2000: 1779–82). Likewise, stem cells of the brain (ectoderm) can differentiate into blood- and muscle cells (mesoderm) (Bjornson et al. 1999: 534–7). Finally, neural stem cells from the brain of adult mice were able to form cells of all three germ layers when injected into blastocysts (Clarke et al. 2000: 1660–63).

Haematopoietic Stem Cells

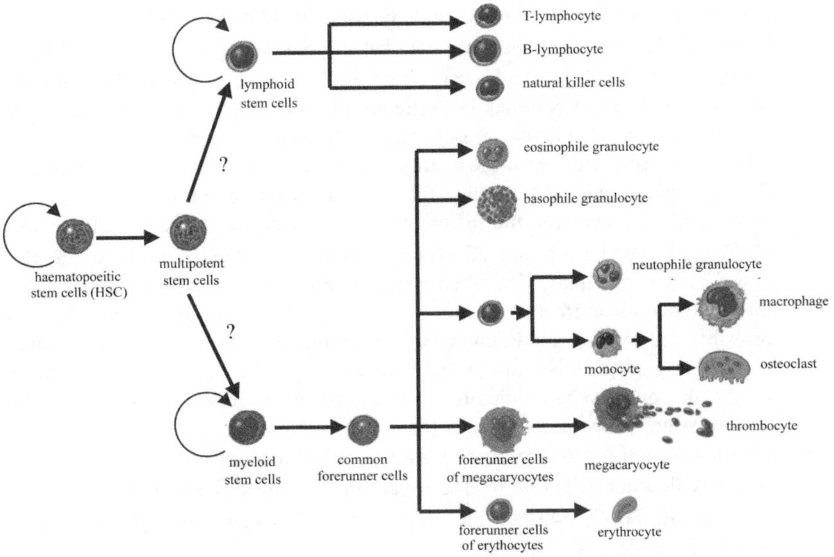

Figure 1 The haematopoietic system. Left, a haematopoietic stem cell (HSC), which produces more HSCs. Their descendants can divide further or produce – as multipotent stem cells – lymphoid or myeloid stem cells, which form all blood cells.

The haematopoietic (blood-forming) stem cells (HSC) of bone marrow are the best-characterized adult stem cells (Fig. 1). They are found not only in bone marrow, but also in the foetal liver and spleen as well as in the blood of the placenta and in the umbilical cord. Under certain experimental conditions, HSC form cell types that are not part of the blood, for example liver cells (Taniguchi et al. 1996: 198–203; Lagasse et al. 2000: 1229–34; Theise et al. 2000: 11–16). Further experiments have suggested that HSC differentiate into an array of cells that integrate into respective tissues; that is, into cells of skeletal muscles, heart muscles, blood vessels and the brain (Gussoni et al. 1999: 390–94; Jackson et al. 2001: 1395–402; Krause et al. 2001: 369–77). A single HSC can differentiate via descendents into cells of all three germ layers. That applies also to a second stem cell type of the bone marrow, the mesenchymal stem cell (see section 'Mesenchymal Stem Cells' below).

Even when many publications allow for a very positive view of therapy with tissue-specific adult stem cells, such as HSC, it must first be shown in most cases whether the results are actually based on the plasticity of these stem cells. A few examples:

- Adult stem cells are very rare, difficult to identify and even more difficult to isolate from the other cells of their respective organs. For this reason, the possibility that there may be several stem cell types in a given tissue cannot at present be excluded. It is also possible that a supposedly well-defined stem cell preparation is in reality a stem cell mixture. As a matter of fact, it was recently shown that the stem cells taken from the muscles of mice that previously had been assumed to be able to form all the important blood cell types had in fact originated in the haematopoietic system (McKinney-Freeman et al. 2002: 1341–6). These HSC that were isolated from muscle were even unable to form colonies in tissue culture that contained muscle cells. This was possible only for the actual muscle stem cells that had been isolated along with the HSC. The explanation for these results was that there are a substantial number of HSC that circulate in the body and thus also may be present in muscles.
- Other work, for example the differentiation of foetal neural stem cells of mice into HSC, could not be reproduced despite extensive studies (Morshead et al. 2002: 268–73). The originally described transformation into blood cells was subsequently interpreted as an artefact of the culture medium. The conditions of the culture medium probably led to the genetic changes (for example, mutations) in the genome of the cells. In any event, it is more probable that non-genetic modifications are responsible for the changes. Such modifications are referred to as epigenetic markings, which will be addressed below (see section 'Epigenetic Problems').
- A further reason for the observed plasticity of some stem cells may well rest on their fusion with other cells that lead to tetraploid cell lines (Terada et al. 2002: 542–5; Ying et al. 2002: 545–8). This is how they broaden their potency and form the observed and described tissues.

The results presented above have intensified the scepticism already raised by many researchers about the pluripotence of adult tissue-specific stem cells (Tsai, Kittappa & McKay 2002: 707–12; Holden & Vogel 2002: 2126–9; D'Amour & Gage 2002: 213–14). In order to establish solid scientific proof of the pluripotence of stem cells, it is therefore necessary to use single, refined and precisely defined cells for future experiments.

Mesenchymal Stem Cells

Mesenchymal stem cells (MSC) (Jiang et al. 2002a: 896–904, and 2000b: 41–9) like HSC can generate offspring of all three germ layers; they yield, for example, all forms of connective and supporting tissues, skeletal musculature, almost all smooth muscle cells, heart musculature and vascular endothelia. MSC have attracted tremendous attention since individual cell lines were cultured over two years ago, and they exhibit important characteristics of pluripotent cells. Individual MSC of mice and rats have been differentiated into a variety of cell types in a culture. An important demonstration for their pluripotence was that after injection into mouse blastocysts they were able to form almost every cell type and also settle in every organ.

Since these cells seem to possess great potential, it is important that they are examined by many laboratories. There are still a multitude of questions when it comes to MSC, such as why MSC have yet to be successfully isolated in persons older than 50 years. One reason might be that adult stem cells themselves are subject to an ageing process (Geiger & Van Zant 2002: 329–33). Then add the common hypothesis that the human body is only designed for a life of about 45 years (see overview in Turker 2000). An extremely important question deals with whether human MSC are at all suitable for therapeutic uses. If they are suitable, then this bone marrow stem cell type would warrant much hope for the future.

Potential and Limits of Therapeutic Uses of Adult Stem Cells

There are a few hurdles that must be cleared before adult stem cells can be employed for therapeutic purposes. The first problem lies in the fact that stem cells, as has already been mentioned, are present in organs only in low numbers. For example, only 1 in 10,000 bone marrow cells are HSC. For adult stem cells to be applied meaningfully, they have to be available in large quantities as well as augmented and reproduced. This leads directly to the second problem of the lack of knowledge about the effective and optimal conditions for adult stem cell culturing and differentiation. This is due to a great extent to the fact that we know almost nothing about the cellular environment of stem cells in situ – the so-called stem cell niche – or about the growth factors that are formed in these niches. Furthermore, we have little knowledge of the behaviour of adult stem cells in an injured tissue and the factors that are necessary for their reproduction and differentiation.

A further problem is the possible rejection of cells by the immune system. Because of the small number of adult stem cells within tissues, they are isolated only with great difficulty, as mentioned above. This is the reason why most bone marrow transplants contain different cell types. However, this is undesirable, since mismatched antigens of the cell membrane (histocompatibility antigens) from donor to recipient can lead a greater number of cells to strengthen immune defences. It is therefore important to improve the methods of purifying haematopoietic stem cells. Additionally, accumulated stem cells colonize blood quicker and more efficiently, which, among other things, reduces the risk of infection (Negrin et al. 2000: 262–71).

HSC from umbilical cord blood will probably be extremely important in the future for disease therapy (Sanchez-Ramos 2002: 880–93). Interestingly, the transplantation of such cells causes no strong defensive reactions (Laughlin et al. 2001: 1815–22). It is presumed that cells of the umbilical blood are less differentiated than cells in the blood of adult organisms and consequently have less immunological effects (Barker et al. 2002: 257–60). A noteworthy advantage of HSC from umbilical blood is that the histocompatibility antigens can be identified and catalogued in advance. However, the number of HSC that can be obtained from the (approximately) 50–150 ml blood of an umbilicus–placenta preparation is very small. It is precisely in this area that serious efforts ought to be undertaken to establish culturing protocols that enable the proliferation and differentiation of HSC. Additionally, it will be extremely important to better understand stem cell niches within organisms (Watt & Hogan 2000; Whetton & Graham 1999: 233–8;). Understanding stem cell niches of model organisms such as the *Drosophilae* fruit fly could be very useful (Spradling, Drummond-Barbosa & Kai 2001: 98–104).

Embryonic Stem Cells

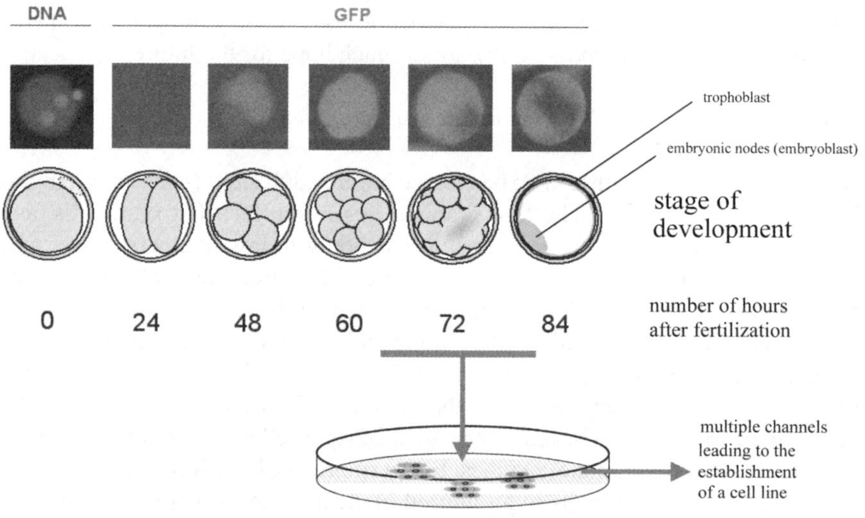

Figure 2 Production of embryonic stem cells (ESC) of mice. In the centre, schematic illustration of development stages. Hour 0: fertilized oocyte; hours 24–72: different stages of division in which the cells cluster close together (morula); hour 84: blastocyst (a hollow embryo) with embryonic knots (embryoblast) and trophoblast (outer hollow sphere). The images show the colouration from Oct-4 about 48 hours after fertilization. The colouration of the fertilized oocyte shows the female and male pronuclei (whose fusion, karyogamy, is still immanent) **and** a small polar body.

Embryonic stem cells (ESC) form the embryonic knots (embryoblast) of the blastocyst (Fig. 2). In humans, there are ESC from about the fourth to the seventh day after fertilization; in mice from about the third to fifth day. Thereafter, the ESC differentiate and form the three germ layers ectoderm, mesoderm and endoderm as the basis of the embryo body.

Potential of Embryonic Stem Cells

In contrast to their rather short developmental period in the embryo, ESC can reproduce indefinitely under certain conditions in culture. Just as within the organism, ESC can also differentiate into a variety of cell types in a culture. Cell lines from ESC (ESC lines) from mice were established more than twenty years ago (Fig. 2). Since then, a wealth of information has been gathered, which facilitates the cultivation and differentiation of ESC lines (see Tables in Boiani & Schoeler 2002; Wobus et al. 2002: 127–56). ESC lines have been able to form different cells of the nervous system, insulin-producing cells, bone cells, cells of the haematopoietic system, endothelial cells, fat cells and varying muscle cell types, for example heart muscle cells.

Human ESC lines were first cultivated successfully in 1998 (Thomson et al. 1998: 1145–7). In his paper, James Thomson showed that human ESC could form benign tumours (teratomas) when injected into mice. These teratomas contained quite complex tissues of ecto-, meso- and endodermic origin. Bone, tooth, hair follicle and lung tissue were found, among others. These results suggest the pluripotence of human ESC. However, they also indicate a possible danger. If ESC or their transformed descendants were to continue in an undifferentiated state, life-threatening tumours (teratocarcinomas) might develop. In order to use ESC lines therapeutically while at the same time excluding the risk of tumour formation, a biological development programme would need to be narrowed by steering it in a desired direction through partial differentiation. It would be ideal to differentiate ESC lines in culture into adult stem cells of a specific potency. This has already been accomplished in mice. It was recently shown that mouse ESC lines produce neural stem cells, which could in turn develop functioning dopaminergic neurons (Kim et al. 2002: 50–56). These cells were capable of significantly reducing Parkinson-type symptoms in rats, which are models for this particular disease. It is true that such successes were already achieved with neural stem cells from foetal, newborn and adult stem cells of mice; however, in these experiments it was not easy to obtain stem cells in any great number. Likewise, it was possible to partially repair spinal cord injuries through the transplantation of ESC from mice (McDonald et al. 1999: 1410–13). Murine ESC were also differentiated into insulin-producing cells that after transplantation were able to produce insulin regulation in diabetics, at least some of the time (Lumelsky et al. 2001: 1389–94).

Likewise Human ESC lines might be shown in the future to be an inexhaustible source for transplantation therapies for the nervous system, liver or pancreas. It must first be shown, however, that the differentiated cells of a model system can ameliorate symptoms of disease. Xenotransplantations, as described in the rat model for Parkinson's disease, would be conceivable in this case between humans and simians. Specifically, I expect that in the not too distant future reports will be published about rhesus monkeys in which diabetes or Parkinson's disease are treated with human cells derived from ESC lines. Together with such functional analyses, it will need to be shown that the transplanted cells integrated into the correct cell colonies. This will be particularly important for nerve- and heart muscle cells, although less so for blood cells.

Problems of Cultivation

In order to preserve their pluripotence, mouse and human ESC lines have so far had to be maintained in media containing serum and nutrient cells. This could be a problem with use in human ESC, because the nutrient cells have come from mice and the serum from calves. This means that zoonoses – infections that can be transmitted from animals to humans – cannot be excluded. A short time ago, however, the cultivation of human ESC with human nutrient cells was described (Richards et al. 2002: 933–6). It remains to be seen whether the tissues employed for nutrient cells (foetal muscle cells, foetal skin cells) are in fact necessary to maintain the pluripotence of the human ESC lines. To avoid zoonoses and, of course, to avoid also the use of human nutrient cells, artificial culturing systems for human ESC lines should be developed. This is no utopian dream; at least for ESC of mice, there has been success in adding to the culture a factor that was produced by nutrient cells (Nichols, Evans & Smith 1990: 1341–8). However, this factor (leukaemia inhibitory factor, LIF) had no influence on human ESC and is consequently unsuitable for such cultures. Even apart from these hurdles, the cultivation and propagation of human ESC lines remains fairly complex.

Before human ESC could be cultured, human embryonic carcinoma cell lines were used to conduct experiments on an early embryonic cell type. In contrast to these cells, ESC lines still have a normal set of chromosomes after more than two years in a culture (Odorico, Kaufmann & Thomson 2001: 193–204). That does not mean, however, that the cultivated ESC lines are free from mutations. As we know from other eukaryotic cells, there is at least one mutation per cell division (Kunkel 1999: 93–4; Kunkel & Bebenek 2000: 497–529). Hence, therapeutic use of cells from old cultures would inevitably entail heightened risk because these cells would carry genetic alterations.

Immunological Problems with the Use of Stem Cells

In the use of embryonic, foetal or adult stem cells, the immunological incompatibility between the stem cell donor and the recipient is a tremendous hurdle. With few exceptions – for instance, with identical twins – their use often leads to a rejection reaction between donor and recipient due to dissimilar histocompatibility antigens. One possibility of avoiding rejection is to fall back on customary procedures, such as the use of immunosuppressives; or, alternatively, combining stem cell transplants from oneself (autologous) and others (allogenic). The problem may also be solved if the recently developed method for rats can be successfully applied (Fandrich et al. 2002: 171–8): in this method, not only entire blastocysts but also cells drawn exclusively from embyroblasts are used to induce tolerance. These cells are relatively free from immunological effect, which may well be due to the fact that the embryo is not acknowledged as foreign during its early development. This advantage could also turn out to be problematic, however, if there is a danger of teratocarcinoma. This is one aspect that has not been addressed in the literature. However, should this prove not to be the case and should we succeed in introducing human HSC derived from ESC lines into the blood system, successive transplantations from differentiated cells or tissues from the same ESC could be carried out.

There are, however, further options for avoiding possible immunological problems. One could culture a high number of different ESC lines of various blastocysts in order to increase the chances of concordance with the histocompatibility antigens of the recipient. Researchers in England have chosen one such approach, in which they hope to cover the better part of the population's histocompatibility antigens with about 300 different ESC lines. There is the further possibility of removing the histocompatibility antigens through homologous recombination of an ESC line in the hope that these cells will not be identified as foreign. This has already proved successful with xenotransplantation. One solution to the immunological questions would only be possible once ESC lineages are developed through therapeutic cloning methods that contain the nucleus of somatic cells. The theory of this method will be examined in the next section.

Therapeutic Clones: Extracting Endogenous ESC Lineages

A form of stem cell therapy is imaginable with cells that are exogenous (allogenic) as well as endogenous (autologous). Both options have advantages and disadvantages.

Allogenic stem cells The advantage of allogenic stem cells is that they can be extracted from a healthy organism. A transplant of allogenic adult or embryonic differentiated stem cells would be practical in a therapy for genetic diseases, for instance. Should the problem of immunological incompatibility between donor and recipient be solvable and, further, should enough stem cells be available, the use of allogenic cells would be an extremely promising option for therapies for a variety of illnesses.

Autologous stem cells Autologous adult stem cells would make it possible to get around the problem of immunological incompatibility. It is certainly questionable whether and to what extent adult stem cells may be taken from a sick person. It is also uncertain how many adult stem cells of a particular type an elderly person might have; much less from a sick elderly person. A further difficulty is that where there is a genetic illness, cells of the patient that carry a harmful mutation will have to be used. Illnesses due to a deficiency of a particular gene product may possibly be treated through the import of appropriate genes. Smuggling genes, for instance, can happen through modified and harmless lentiviruses that are able to infect stem cells. Such an infection would be carried out in vitro before being transferred to the recipient (see Overview in Woods, Ooka & Karlsson 2002: 563–9). However, there are also multiple genetic problems for which such a gene transfer would be of no assistance. For example, a symptom profile could be created such that a mutation in a gene leads to a defective protein that in turn impairs cell function. Furthermore, it is not possible at the moment to make such insertions, much less regulate the quantity of cultured proteins placed inside a cell. However, exactly this is often what is essential in the physiological context. It would harm the body in the long run if, for instance, the genetically modified cells were to constantly produce insulin.

The only way out in such cases would be to correct the genetic defect in the stem cell before transplantation through so-called homologous recombination, which means trading the specified mutant gene sequences for normal DNA sequences. In this way, the proper regulation of the gene would remain safeguarded. However, at the moment this procedure is not practicable with adult stem cells. The homologous recombination method was established for ESC lines – at least, for mouse ESC – and for these it is quite useful. Human ESC are available only until the seventh day of development. As such, endogenous, individual ESC lines (autologous ESC), from which homologous recombination could be eventually accomplished, cannot be produced. Autologous human ESC can be generated only through the process of so-called therapeutic cloning, which will be discussed in the next section.

Methods

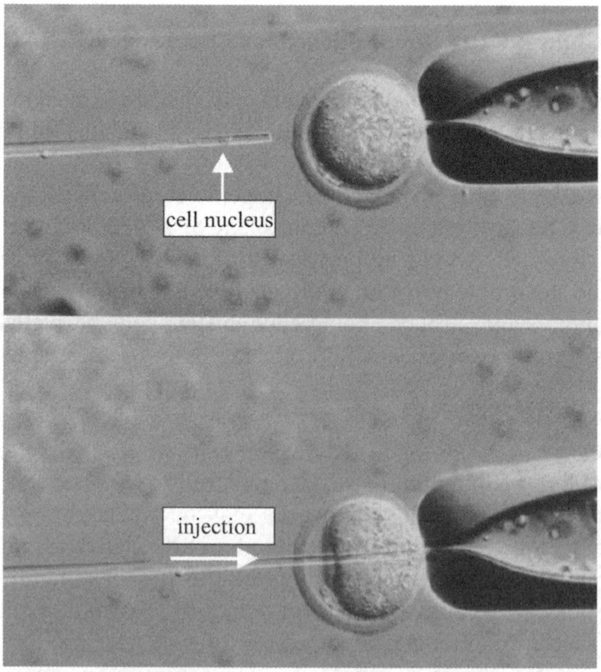

Figure 3. Transfer of a cell nucleus of a mouse somatic cell into an enucleated mouse oocyte.

The following approaches would be possible, in principle, in order to draw endogenous, individual ESC-equivalent cells or cell lines. For each approach, one would use and experiment with the diploid cell nucleus from differentiated somatic cells or the entire cells from the patient as raw material to produce ESC lines or ESC-similar cells and cell lines. In the first place, there would be different ways to bring the cell nucleus back to its full potential. A procedure that has already been successfully conducted in a series of animal experiments is the nuclear transfer of somatic cells (NTSC) in cored oocytes (egg cells; see Fig. 3) and their subsequent further development in culture into blastocysts.

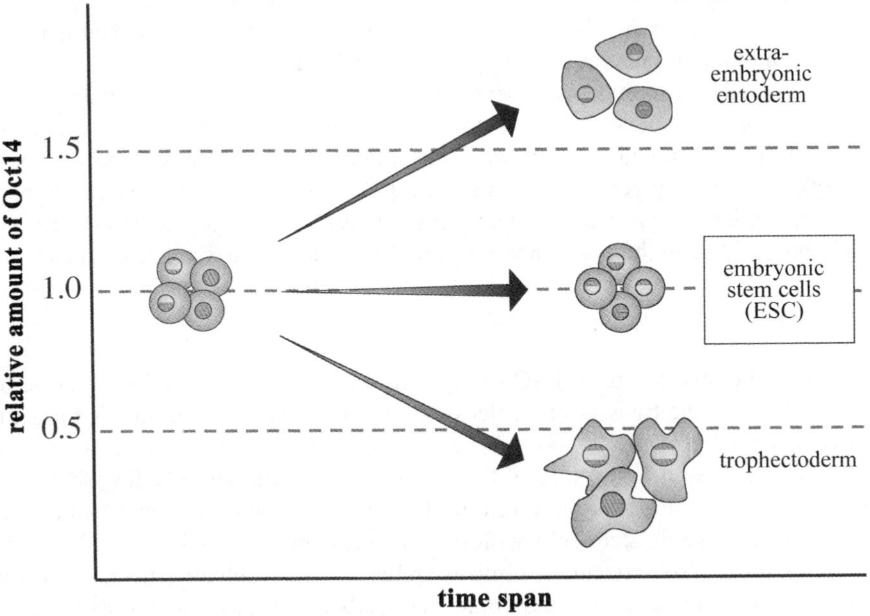

Figure 4. Oct-4 and pluripotence. As long as the Oct-4 protein is in a determined relative quantity, a cell retains its embryonic stem cell status. With differentiation, its pluripotence is lost.

ESC lines have already been successfully derived from blastocysts resulting from NTSC in mice (Munsie et al. 2000: 989–92; Wakayama et al. 2001: 740–43). It remains to be seen why such experiments are successful, even though in most cases the blastocysts are not viable (Boiani et al. 2002: 1209–19). What is important here is the protein product of the so-called Oct-4 gene, which is essential for the maintenance of ESC pluripotence (Pesce & Schöler 2000: 452–7, and 2001: 271–6). Clearly only a particular amount of Oct-4 is formed by pluripotent ESC (Fig. 4). A difference of ± 50% has dramatic consequences because then the ESC differentiate and lose their pluripotence (Niwa, Miyazaki & Smith 2000: 372–6; Yoshimizu et al. 1999: 675–84; Yeom et al. 1996: 881–94).

Because of the genome quality of somatic cells from which the cell nucleus is removed, it would be important to produce several ESC lines through nucleus transfer in order to decide which would be best for later use. Because of the inadequate DNA quality of somatic cells and the various packaging of DNA through chromatin proteins, the quality of the created cell lines cannot be determined in advance. A great advantage of cell lines that have been created through nucleus transfer would be that they could be thoroughly examined and selected for their suitability (for example, their ability to form a particular cell type) in a culture before being used in stem cell therapy. A further advantage would be that this examination would need to be conducted with only a part of the cell of such a line. The other part could be preserved in liquid nitrogen. If a line should later prove itself suitable, the frozen material could be used. These procedures would prevent an established cell line from accumulating mutations due to prolonged cultivation.

In conventional animal experiments, employing nuclear transfer methods requires the use of natural oocytes. Their extraction is extremely complex and in humans it would be in combination with to a very unpleasant procedure. It now appears possible, however, to generate oocytes from ESC in culture. This has recently been done with mice (Hübner et al. 2003: 1251–6). With the help of such oocytes, we might possibly be in the position to generate ESC lines through nuclear transfer.

Reprogramming

In order to be able to create ESC lines as described above, it would be necessary to reprogramme the transferred nucleus of a matured somatic cell; that is to say, to reset its genetic programme to an earlier starting point in embryonic development. However, because the resulting ESC lines would be required only for therapeutic purposes, it is not necessary to return to the very beginning. In place of an oocyte, eventually embryonic stem cells without nuclei (cytoplasts) could be used in order to reprogramme a somatic nucleus into an embryonic stem cell nucleus. Experiments that have fused somatic and embryonic stem cells of a mouse have already shown that ESC are able to alter the additional nucleus such that it contains characteristics of natural ESC nuclei. An important task would be to determine which cellular factors are responsible for reprogramming somatic nuclei. That would then probably lead to the development of a production method for endogenous, individual ESC lines without the use of oocytes and embryonic cells.

Reproductive Clones

Nuclear transfer for the creation of viable organisms is referred to as reproductive cloning. Not only are there objections against reproductive cloning based on ethics, but there are numerous biological reasons as well. Currently, the cloning efficiency – the percentage of organisms born that survive nuclear transfer into oocytes – is somewhere around 3 to 5 per cent within a few animal species; within most species, it is significantly lower. This is certainly to be considered progress, but even then it may well be impossible either to avoid the death of embryos and foetuses or to estimate whether or not the transferred nucleus carries genetic defects. Whether the famous cloned sheep Dolly suffered from arthritis due to a genetic defect has yet to be resolved, much less at what state and how the 276 'experimental failures' died preceding Dolly's birth (Wilmut et al. 1997: 810–13). As most of the protagonists of reproductive cloning are unaware or do not perceive this as much of a problem, it will certainly be important, through further animal experiments, to reveal that creating viable organisms through reproductive cloning is purely a matter of statistical chance and is unpredictable. There are numerous grounds as to why nuclei and somatic cells are inappropriate for cloning organisms that are free from threatening mutations. Some of the reasons will be laid out in the next section.

Problems with Cloning

The biological programme for development is controlled not only by genetic but also by epigenetic factors. Under genetic controls, the whole course of events is understood as being determined directly through genes (as well as through the gene-coded proteins). A gene can function only when the DNA sequence of the genome is intact. Epigenetic controls encompass every interaction between cell parts or between cells that contribute to development, but they are genetically prescribed only indirectly. Modifications and packaging of genomes are particularly epigenetically active (externally recognizable on chromatin, the stainable components of the nucleus that consist of DNA, histons and non-histoproteins). Epigenetic controls take effect only if defects in the chromatin are not too great. Where modifications or the packaging of the genome are disturbed, it is possible for tumours to form.

Genetic Problems

As with every long-living, multi-celled organism, the human body is subject to external mutagenic agents, the effects of which accumulate throughout its life. The list of such factors includes, for example, UV and ionized background radiation; chemical mutagens such as aflatoxin, benzene and N-nitrosamine; and infection with cancer-causing viruses. Together with these exogenous dangers, there are a number of dangers that live within the organism itself: with every cell division, DNA is damaged, which can be a starting point for a tumour if mutations are not repaired. In May 2000, there were 21,591 known mutations in more than 1000 human genes that are responsible for a wide variety of problems (Fig. 5) (Antonarakis, Krawczak & Cooper 2000: 173–8). It can be assumed that human cells experience a multiplicity of DNA premutations daily. We speak of premutations when there is a chance that the changes will be corrected. However, as DNA repair does not work perfectly, a few premutations are the source for spontaneously arising mutations. Both the occasional appearance of non-repaired damaged nucleotides and faulty reading during replication can lead to tumours and other illnesses. Changes to the genome occur even during embryonic development. For example, in blood from healthy newborns, highly sensitive methods have verified an exchange of chromosome fragments that could induce tumours (Mori et al. 2002: 8242–7).

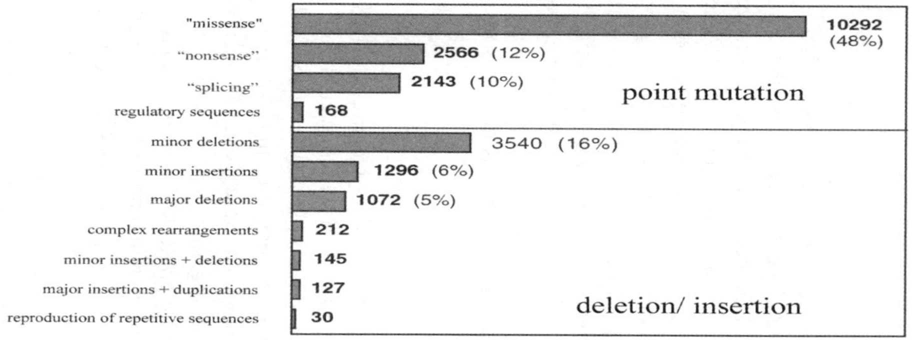

Figure 5 Disease-causing mutations in human genomes. A spectrum of different mutations, separated by type and frequency. At the time of the analysis, there were in total 21,591 known mutations in 1039 genes (see Antonarakis, Krawczak & Cooper 2000: 173–8).

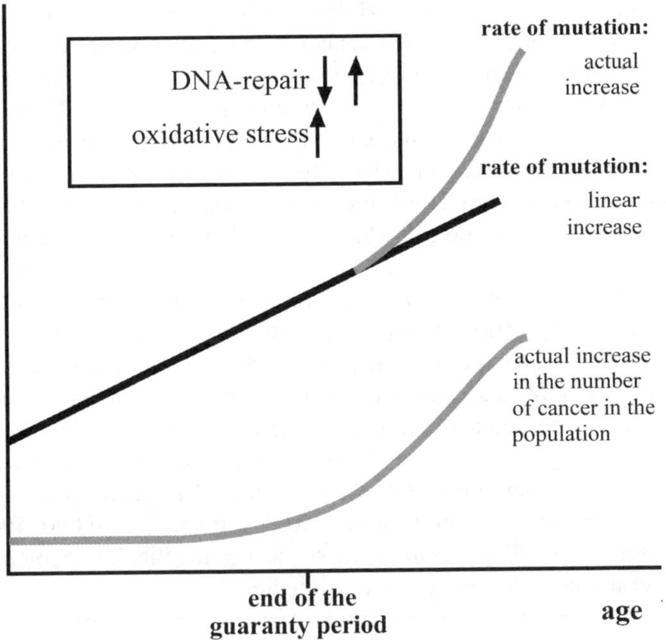

Figure 6 Correlation of mutation rate and cancer with increasing age. If several mutations have taken place, there is an exponential increase of cancer (see Turker 2000).

Premutations are undone through precise and highly efficient repair systems. Therefore, there is a high probability that no tumours develop until a person is 45 years old (Turker 2000). Thereafter, the 'warranty has run out', and both the frequency of mutations and the probability of tumours developing increases rapidly (Fig. 6).

Stem cell and cloning experts give almost no consideration to the destructive consequences of mutations. This is completely incomprehensible, because one must be informed about the different mutation types in order to recognize which dangers the cloned organisms would be exposed to. The following mutations and processes play a role in connection with this.

Changes through punctuated mutations DNA-punctuated mutations can be traced largely to three main causes: unstable N-glycosyl bonds, a deamination of methylated DNA and oxidative stress (overview in Lindahl 1993: 709–15). Mutations can further produce repetitive genomic segments through recombination. Transitions from cytosine (C) to thymine (T) cause about a third of all punctuated mutations found in genetically transmitted human diseases (Cooper & Youssoufian 1988: 151–5). These rather complex problems are described in Box 2 and Table 1.

Transcription-coupled DNA repair The enzyme RNA-polymerase II transfers DNA into mRNAs (transcription) that are translated ultimately into proteins (translation). More than fifteen years ago, it was established that transcribed and active genes are repaired far faster than inactive genes (Svejstrup 2002: 1151–2). A result is that mutations occur in inactive genes more frequently than in active genes. This presents no problem if the former remain inactive. So it is no problem if, for example, genes that are expressed only in brain cells mutate into muscle cells: there, they would be unnecessary and remain turned off, which is why they can cause no harm.

Mutations through recombination of repetitive genome segments Monogenetic sicknesses are usually caused by specific mutations within a defined gene. Such mutations can usually be traced back to mistakes during DNA replication. Moreover, there are diseases that are caused by recombinations of genomic regions. The primary source is gene duplication; repetitive genome sequences (RGS) result from this process. Repetitions of original genomic regions are referred to as paralogue genomic regions and they form RGS. An exchange of fragments can occur among the RGS of one or several chromosomes. RGS are usually 10,000–400,000 base pairs long with at least 97 per cent of the sequences identical, thereby presenting a suitable substrate for a homologous recombination.

Box 2:

From Premutations to Punctuated Mutations

Premutations: One speaks of premutations if there is a chance that the changes can be repaired before they manifest as mutations (compare Table 1). Spontaneously occurring mutations can usually be traced back to faulty DNA repair. This, along with erroneous reading during replication, can certainly lead to tumour formation.

Sources of Defects and Repair Possibilities

Labile N-Glycosyl bonding: All biological macromolecules are unstable and decompose with time. Nucleic acids (DNA and RNA) decompose in solution; RNA is particularly unstable. Through the presence of a hydroxyl group in the 2 position of ribose, its phosphodiesther bond is particularly sensitive to hydrolysis. The phosphodiesther bonds of DNA are far more stable, although this is at the cost of the stability of the n-glycosyl bonds, through which sugar (deoxyribose) and bases are combined. In metabolically active cells, DNA is present in a completely hydrated form and one assumes that they lose bases as quickly as they do in solution. Within the cell, the base-free spots of DNA are repaired with extreme efficiency by a variety of enzymes.
Deamination of Methylated DNA: The hydrolytic transformation from cytosine into uracil at a neutral pH value is caused by the direct deamination

through hydrolysis. 5-methylcytosine loses amino groups about three to four times faster than cytosine (C) does, so that the deamination of 5-methylcytosine presents an important source of mutation. In mammals, cytosine is frequently methylated if it is in the vicinity of guanine in the DNA strand (so-called CG dinucleotide). Particularly this methylation has an influence on the activity of genes (there is less methylation in transcriptionally active genes than in inactive ones). The problem is not so much in the loss of amino groups as in their repair. If cytosine is deaminated within cells, uracil results (U), which will be removed by uracil-DNA-glycosylase, whereupon the base-free location is corrected efficiently. This glycosylase cannot use deaminated 5-methylcytosine (or Thymine, T) as substrate. Hence, in mammals, faulty guanine–thymine (G–T) base pairings are repaired by rather slow correcting enzymes. The increased rate of deaminations from 5-methylcytosine as well as the relatively slow repair of faulty G–T base pairs result in CG sequences showing an approximately 40-times higher mutation rate than sequences from other dinucleotides. It may be that these transitions from C to T are responsible for about a third of all point mutations that lead to congenital human diseases. The mutation frequency of CG dinucleotides from TG depends upon the particular gene. Comparing human genes with one another, for example, in b-globin- and HPRT genes, less than 10% of CG dinucleotides mutate, whereas in ADA genes it is 50% (Sharpless & DePinho 2002).

Oxidative Stress: During normal metabolism, aerobically growing cells are exposed to active oxygen that can be a major cause of endogenous damage. A damaged base that can lead to a mutation is 8-hydroxyl guanine. Hydroxyl guanine is produced and acted upon primarily by hydroxyl radicals that at this point pair it with adenine rather than with cytosine. This reaction leads to mutations during replication if a DNA glycosylase fails to splice of the damaged sequence in good time. There are a whole series of possible causes for mutations, whose course has yet to be investigated in detail. An example of the potential for endogenous damage is the formation of H_2O_2 through stimulated polymorphic nuclear leucocytes and monocytes. Additionally, tumours can form considerable quantities of H_2O_2. These very potent means of oxidation can damage DNA despite endogenous catalysis.

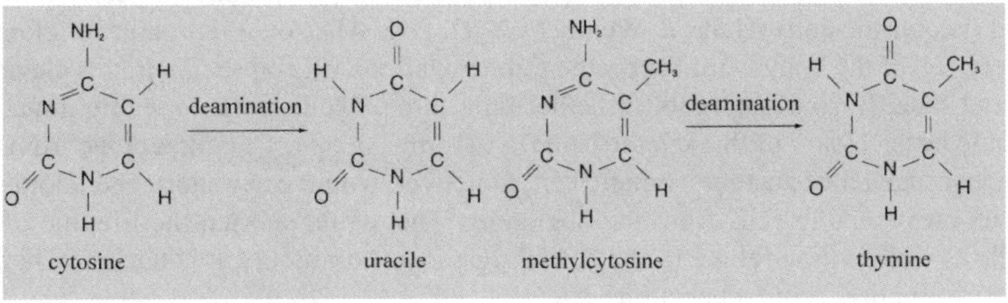

Mutations that result from ageing There are different theories regarding the ageing process that are not mutually exclusive (Guarente & Kenyon 2000: 255–62). One long-discussed theory states that, with increasing age, there is a decrease in DNA repair activity and an accompanying increased incidence of DNA damage (Sharpless & Depinho 2002: 9–12). Procedures that damage DNA, such as radiation and chemotherapy, can induce processes that resemble natural ageing. Examples are reduced wound healing, early menopause, hair loss and premature senility. Often genes are affected whose protein products detect DNA damage and/or are involved in DNA repair. Further, there is a connection between the shortening of chromosome ends (telomeres) and cell age. Because telomeres are shortened by each cell division, one speaks of them in connection to a life clock. A third theory makes a connection between oxidative stress, metabolism and age. There are numerous data from animal models that support this theory: mutations – for example, that reduce glucose metabolism – lengthen the lifespan of many animal species. One assumes that a lower metabolism leads to less toxic forms of oxygen. Protein p53 may play a key role in each of the three processes. It appears, on the one hand, to supress existing tumours, and, on the other hand, to restrict the repair and regeneration of normal cells (Sharpless & Depinho 2002: 9–12). Mice that received a hyperactive p53 variant into the germ line were immune to cancer, but aged faster. In this regard, their recovery was like that of animals that had shown defective DNA repair or that had only short telomeres. In short, p53 appears to minimise the development of new tumours, but at the cost of the repair and regeneration of normal tissue.

The above processes could have serious consequences for a cloned organism; that is, for an organism that was generated by the transfer of a cell nucleus from a somatic cell into an oocyte. The clone, for example, suspends the inactive status of cell-specific genes. If an organism were then to be generated from the nucleus of a muscle cell, the many of the inactivated genes (for example, genes for the development of specific cells required by the brain) in the nucleus would be reactivated. Should mutations appear in these genes, it might lead to complications in the developing tissues and organs (for example, brain cells). Such genes can form defective proteins, be imported into the wrong cells, or be read in non-physiological masses. Because the human body has more than 200 different cell types, it is easy to see what would happen if all the inert muscle cell genes in the entire body were reactivated. Existing mutations need not immediately cause problems. In human cells, for example, four to six mutations are necessary to produce an early tumour cell (neoplastic cell) (Hahn & Weinberg 2002: 331–41). As in reproductive cloning every cell of the body would carry the same mutations, all cells begin in this elevated initial state. It is unforeseeable whether four, three, two or only one more mutation would be necessary to 'breach the levee' and form a neoplastic cell. A clone from the nuclear transfer of an adult somatic cell, moreover, would carry shortened telomeres in its own somatic cells from the beginning. That could shorten the lifetime of its cells as well as the lifetime of the entire organism. Admittedly, it is unclear whether this assumption is in fact accurate.

Table 1 **Table of endogenous DNA lesions in human cells and the possible means of punctuated mutation. Full version in Lindahl 1993.**

Lesions/ premutations	**Type of lesions and mutation formation**	**Number of modifications and premutations per cell per day**	**Number of modifications and premutations that remain in normal cells**
Uracil	Deamination of cytosine	400	1
Thymine	Deamination of 5-methylcytosine	30	10–20
Hypoxanthine	Deamination of adenine	10	1
8-Oxoguanine	Oxidation of guanine	1000	1
Formamido-Pyrimidine	Oxidation of guanine	200	5
Thymine glycol and similar oxid. pyrimidine	Oxidation of pyrimidine	500	5
Ethyl-Cytosine	Lipid peroxidation of cytosine	200	5
Ethyl-Adenine	Lipid peroxidation of adenine	200	5
3-Methyl-Adenine	SAM-Methylation of adenine	600	5
7-Methyl-Guanine	SAM-Methylation of Guanine	4000	3000
O^6-Methyl-Guanine	Through endogenous nitrosamine	200	1
Without base	Hydrolysis	9000	5

Despite these risks for the somatic cell genome, mutations are no problem for germ line cells. Apparently, these have particular mechanisms at their disposal that put them in a position to generate sperm or oocytes of a higher genome quality over many years. Possible reasons for this will not be discussed at this time; even cells of a higher genomic quality are entirely unsuited to cloning because there are serious epigenetic problems, which are presented next.

Epigenetic Problems

Germ cells and imprinting Germ line development connects individuals of a species, and for this reason it is potentially immortal. In every generation, oocytes and spermatozoa are formed whose union is the starting point of a new organism. In a few vertebrates, the oocyte is also able to create an organism without sperm. This is referred to as parthenogenesis and can occur in reptiles, birds, fish and amphibians. These form from non-inseminated oocytes such that only the female genome contributes to the organism's development. Additionally, some mammals (for example, mice, rabbits and pigs) can occasionally form embryos parthenogenetically, but they die during embryonic development. Experimentally, mammal embryos have been produced that are of purely male (androgenetic) or purely female (gynogenetic) origin. For this, either two female (maternal) or two male (paternal) pronuclei were brought together through transplantation into an enucleated oocyte. Embryonic development is then controlled by the genetic information of only one sex. In all three cases, however, the embryos die because whereas the female and the male genome certainly contain the same genes, some of those genes' functions differ based on their origin (male or female).

If the function of a gene depends on its sex, this must have an epigenetic cause described as genetic marking or imprinting. Imprinting probably functions so that certain genes are read – that is, expressed – from only the maternal or the paternal genome. Imprinting is based on diverse methylation of the maternal and paternal genes. Upon fusion of egg and sperm, the sex-specific methylation pattern unites and is later repeated from cell division to cell division.

Imprinting would have significant relevance for reproductive cloning: if cell nuclei from either germ cells or their forerunners were employed for cloning, the resulting embryo would carry only the marking of the maternal or paternal genomes. The very early germ cells, the original germ cells, produced during the development of an organism – like all other cells – have maternal and paternal markings. As they develop, however, these markings are reset; that is, the old are removed and, according to sex, are replaced by the maternal or paternal markings. The result is that embryos that are attempts to clone from germ cells die for similar reasons as the above-mentioned androgenetic, gynogenetic or parthenogenetic mammal embryos (Mori et al. 2002: 8242–7).

A further problem would be that the transfer of the markings in germ cells and somatic cells is often imprecise. As has already been discussed with regard to 'sleeping mutations', this is irrelevant because epigenetic markings play no role in most cells of the organism. If, however, a cell nucleus were to be used for reproductive cloning, a faulty reading during early development could be extremely problematic.

Reprogramming Along with methylation, genome packaging must be changed if cloning via somatic cell nuclei is to be successful. Many genes that were active in their respective somatic cells need to be turned off, while others that were inactive need to be turned back on, so that an embryo can develop. Epigenetic reprogramming during normal development and during the cloning process is among the most interesting themes of molecular biology at this time (Li 2002: 662–73). It is still unknown, though, how the old proteins and modifications are replaced with the new.

In any event, it is to be expected that, based on these epigenetic phenomena, what has already been discussed above will also apply to a cloned organism: the faulty packaging of a genome and its resulting defective activation or deactivation by genes would have far-reaching, but unforeseeable, consequences. In short, based on the genetic and epigenetic problems presented, it is very probable that organisms produced through nuclear transfer may well exhibit damage that becomes evident either sooner in embryonic development or perhaps only later, which is to say certainly at some time in the adult organism.

Adult Stem Cell Nuclei and Cloning

Could nuclei from adult stem cells eventually prove more suitable for cloning organisms than nuclei from differentiated, matured somatic cells? Even if there is not the same wealth of information for the former as for the latter, there is no reason to assume that the same genetic and epigenetic problems could not arise. In fact, there is increasing indication, for example, that adult stem cells are also subject to an ageing process (Geiger & Van Zant 2002: 329–33).

Even nuclei of embryonic stem cells would not be good for cloning organisms. Although they represent an extremely early stage of development and thereby have an epigenetic programme that should be quite similar to the programme of the inseminated egg cell, experiments with cloned mice show that many genes in the animals' organs were read incorrectly. Irrespective of whether the nucleus of a somatic cell or an ESC is used to clone, about 1 in 25 will be incorrectly expressed (Humpherys et al. 2002: 12889–94). This number provides very strong evidence, because in the study cited more than 10,000 genes were investigated simultaneously. That means that in every organ of a clone, hundreds of genes will be incorrectly expressed. This is probably due to the fact that at the beginning of embryonic development, important regulatory key genes, such as the Oct-4 gene, could not be read correctly (Boiani et al. 2002: 1209–19).

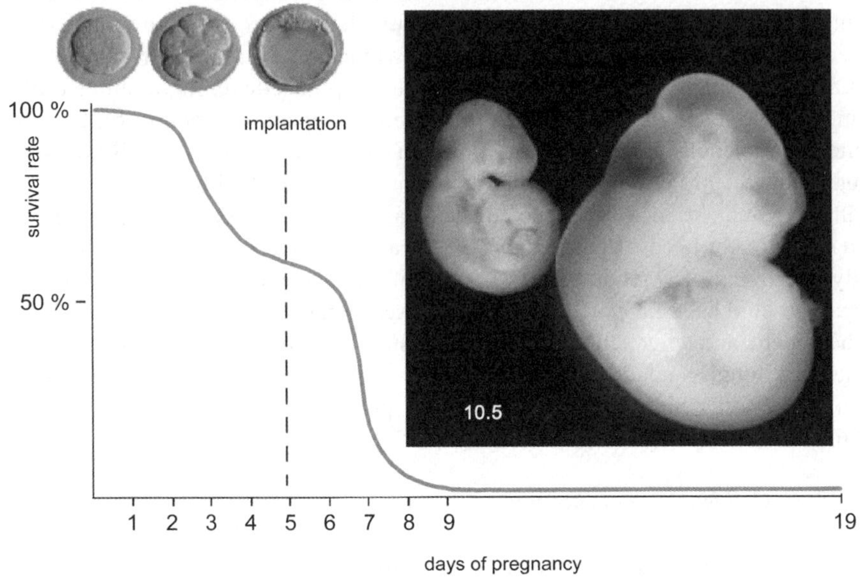

Figure 7 The reproductive cloning of mice. Survival rate of embryos and foetuses during pregnancy. Immediately after implantation, only a few embryos are capable of further development. Just 10 days after fertilization, when most of the foetuses have already died, the few surviving foetuses have serious problems. The picture on the right shows two ten-and-a-half days old foetuses. The one on the left was cloned; the one on the right is the result of normal fertilization.

Depending on the genes affected, the clones will die either as embryos or as foetuses. In a few instances (even among the 3 to 5 per cent of survivors), the problems will be transmitted during the development from cell to cell (Fig. 7). The fact that changes that are not initially evident can have dramatic consequences is later shown in the obese mice that are often produced in the cloning process (Tamashiro et al. 2002: 262–7). Up to about the tenth week after birth, these mouse clones have a normal body weight that increases rather dramatically thereafter. The pairing of two fat-bodied mice leads to an interesting result: although the parents were extremely heavy, the offspring, rather than being even fatter, were instead as slender as normal mice. This result clearly shows that the new packaging of the genome was faulty during cloning. Only if this is modified once again can the normal development programme run. In addition, the genes whose faulty reading led to the obesity were correctly repackaged. This happened during gametogenesis; that is, during the formation of sperm and egg cells. In the example mentioned, only in the subsequent generation was it possible for all the genes to be correctly read and for the mice to develop a normal body weight. It remains to be seen, however, whether the obese mice or the animals of the next generation will develop tumours or other problems later in life.

The findings of the animal experiments presented above make it clear that these expected problems from reproductive cloning would be neither foreseeable nor necessarily immediately apparent. Whether every tenth, twenty-fifth or hundredth gene would be incorrectly read is not that important. With presumably 66,000 genes in the human genome, that would in any case amount to a lot of affected genes. The magnitude of the resulting problems will be made clear through future animal experiments.

Bibliography

Aboody, K.S., et al. (2000) 'Neural stem cells display extensive tropism for pathology in adult brain: Evidence from intracranial gliomas', *Proceedings of the National Academy of Science USA*, **97**, 12846–51 [DOI: 10.1073/pnas.97.23.12846]

Antonarakis, S.E., **Krawczak, M.**, and **Cooper, D.N.** (2000) 'Disease-causing mutations in the human genome', *European Journal of Pediatrics*, **159**, Supplement 3, 173–8 [DOI: 10.1007/PL00014395]

Barker, J.N., et al. (2002) 'Searching for unrelated donor hematopoietic stem cells: Availability and speed of umbilical cord blood versus bone marrow', *Biology of Blood and Marrow Transplantation*, **8**, 257–60 [PubMed: 12064362] [DOI: 10.1053/ bbmt.2002.v8.pm12064362]

Bjornson, C.R., et al. (1999) 'Turning brain into blood: A hematopoetic fate adopted by adult neural stem cells in vivo', *Science*, **283**, 534–7 [PubMed: 9915700] [DOI: 10.1126/science.283.5401.534]

Boiani, M., and **Schöler, H.R.** (2002) 'Determinants of pluripotency in mammals', in *Principles of Cloning,* eds R. Lanza, J. Cibelli and M. West, San Diego: Academic Press, pp. 109–52

Boiani, M., et al. (2002) '-4 Distribution and level in mouse clones: Consequences for pluripotency', *Genes and Development*, **16**, 1209–19 [PubMed: 12023300] [DOI: 10.1101/gad.966002]

Clarke, D.L., et al. (2000) 'Generalized potential of adult neural stem cells', *Science*, **288**, 1660–63 [PubMed: 10834848] [DOI: 10.1126/science.288.5471.1660]

Cooper, D.N., and **Youssoufian, H.** (1988) 'The CpG dinucleotide and human genetic disease', *Human Genetics*, **78**, 151–5 [PubMed: 3338800] [DOI: 10.1007/ BF00278187]

D'Amour, K.A., and **Gage, F.H.** (2002) 'Are somatic stem cells pluripotent or lineage restricted?',*Nature Medicine*, **8**, 213–14 [PubMed: 11875484] [DOI: 10.1038/ nm0302-213]

Fandrich, F., et al. (2002) 'Preimplantation-stage stem cells induce long-term allogeneic graft acceptance without supplementary host conditioning', *Nature Medicine*, **8**, 171–8 [PubMed: 11821902] [DOI: 10.1038/nm0202-171]

Geiger, H., and **Van Zant, G.** (2002) 'The aging of lympho-hematopoietic stem cells', *Nature Immunology*, **3**, 329–33 [PubMed: 11919569] [DOI: 10.1038/ ni0402-329]

Guarente, L., and **Kenyon, C.** (2000) 'Genetic pathways that regulate ageing in model organisms', *Nature*, **408**, 255–62 [PubMed: 11089983] [DOI: 10.1038/35041700]

Gussoni, E., et al. (1999) 'Dystrophin expression in the mdx mouse restored by stem cell transplantation', *Nature*, **401**, 390–94 [PubMed: 10517639] [DOI: 10.1038/43922]

Hahn, W.C.. and **Weinberg, R.A.** (2002) 'Modeling the molecular circuitry of cancer', *Nature Reviews Cancer*, **2**, 331–41 [PubMed: 12044009] [DOI: 10.1038/nrc795]

Holden, C., and **Vogel, G.** (2002) 'Plasticity: Time for a reappraisal?', *Science*, **296**, 2126–9 [PubMed: 12077383] [DOI: 10.1126/science.296.5576.2126]

Hübner, R., et al. (2003) 'Derivation of oocytes from mouse embryonic stem cells', *Science*, **300**, 1251–6 [DOI: 10.1126/science.1083452]

Humpherys, D., et al. (2002) 'Abnormal gene expression in cloned mice derived from embryonic stem cell and cumulus cell nuclei', *Proceedings of the National Academy of Science USA*, **99**, 12889–94 [DOI: 10.1073/pnas.192433399]

Jackson, K.A., et al. (2001) 'Regeneration of ischemic cardiac muscle and vascular endothelium by adult stem cells', *Journal of Clinical Investigation*, **107**, 1395–402 [PubMed: 11390421]

Jiang, Y., et al. (2002a) 'Multipotent progenitor cells can be isolated from postnatal murine bone marrow, muscle, and brain', *Experimental Hematology*, **30**, 896–904 [DOI: 10.1016/S0301-472X%2802%2900869-X]

Jiang, Y., et al. (2002b) 'Pluripotency of mesenchymal stem cells derived from adult marrow', *Nature*, **418**, 41–9 [DOI: 10.1038/nature00870]

Kim, J.H., et al. (2002) 'Dopamine neurons derived from embryonic stem cells function in an animal model of Parkinson's disease', *Nature*, **418**, 50–56 [PubMed: 12077607] [DOI: 10.1038/nature00900]

Kirschstein, R., and **Skirboll, L.R.** (2001) 'Stem cells: Scientific progress and future directions', National Institute of Health (NIH), Bethesda

Krause, D.S., et al. (2001) 'Multi-organ, multi-lineage engraftment by a single bone marrow-derived stem cell', *Cell*, **105**, 369–77 [PubMed: 11348593] [DOI: 10.1016/S0092-8674%2801%2900328-2]

Kunkel, T.A. (1999) 'The high cost of living', *Trends in Genetics*, **15**, 93–4 [PubMed: 10203802] [DOI: 10.1016/S0168-9525%2898%2901664-3]

Kunkel, T.A., and **Bebenek, K.** (2000) 'DNA replication fidelity', *Annual Review of Biochemistry*, **69**, 497–529 [PubMed: 10966467] [DOI: 10.1146/annurev.biochem.69.1.497]

Lagasse, E., et al. (2000) 'Purified hematopoietic stem cells can differentiate into hepatocytes in vivo', *Nature Medicine*, **6**, 1229–34 [PubMed: 11062533] [DOI: 10.1038/81326]

Laughlin, M.J., et al. (2001) 'Hematopoietic engraftment and survival in adult recipients of umbilical-cord blood from unrelated donors', *The New England Journal of Medicine*, **344**, 1815–22 [PubMed: 11407342] [DOI: 10.1056/NEJM200106143442402]

Li, E. (2002) 'Chromatin modification and epigenetic reprogramming in mammalian development', *Nature Reviews Genetics*, **3**, 662–73 [PubMed: 12209141] [DOI: 10.1038/nrg887]

Lindahl, T. (1993) 'Instability and decay of the primary structure of DNA', *Nature*, **362**, 709–15 [PubMed: 8469282] [DOI: 10.1038/362709a0]

Lumelsky, N., et al. (2001) 'Differentiation of embryonic stem cells to insulin-secreting structures similar to pancreatic islets', *Science*, **292**, 1389–94 [PubMed: 11326082] [DOI: 10.1126/science.1058866]

McDonald, J.W., et al. (1999) 'Transplanted embryonic stem cells survive, differentiate and promote recovery in injured rat spinal cord', *Nature Medicine*, **5**, 1410–13 [PubMed: 10581084] [DOI: 10.1038/70986]

McKinney-Freeman, S.L., et al. (2002) 'Muscle-derived hematopoietic stem cells are hematopoietic in origin', *Proceedings of the National Academy of Science USA*, **99**, 1341–6 [DOI: 10.1073/pnas.032438799]

Mezey, E., et al. (2000) 'Turning blood into brain: Cells bearing neural antigens generated in vivo from bone marrow', *Science*, **290**, 1779–82 [PubMed: 11099419] [DOI: 10.1126/science.290.5497.1779]

Mori, H., et al. (2002) 'Chromosome translocation and covert leukemic clones are generated during normal fetal development', *Proceedings of the National Academy of Science USA*, **99**, 8242–7 [DOI: 10.1073/pnas.112218799]

Morshead, C.M., et al. (2002) 'Hematopoietic competence is a rare property of neural stem cells that may depend on genetic and epigenetic alterations,' *Nature Medicine*, **8**, 268–73 [PubMed: 11875498] [DOI: 10.1038/nm0302-268]

Munsie, M.J., et al. (2000) 'Isolation of pluripotent embryonic stem cells from reprogrammed adult mouse somatic cell nuclei,' *Current Biology*, **10**, 989–92 [PubMed: 10985386] [DOI: 10.1016/S0960-9822%2800%2900648-5]

Negrin, R.S., et al. (2000) 'Transplantation of highly purified CD 34+Thy-1+ hematopoietic stem cells in patients with metastatic breast cancer', *Biology of Blood and Marrow Transplantation*, **6**, 262–71 [PubMed: 10871151] [DOI: 10.1016/S1083-8791%2800%2970008-5]

Nichols, J., **Evans, E.P.,** and **Smith, A.G.** (1990) '*Establishment of Germ-Line-Competent Embryonic Stem* (ES) cells using differentiation inhibiting activity', *Development*, 110, 1341–8

Niwa, H., **Miyazaki, J.**, and **Smith, A.G.** (2000) 'Quantitative expression of Oct-3/4 defines differentiation, dedifferentiation or self-renewal of ES cells,' *Nature Genetics*, **24**, 372–6 [PubMed: 10742100] [DOI: 10.1038/74199]

Noble, M. (2000a) 'Can neural stem cells be used as therapeutic vehicles in the treatment of brain tumors?', *Nature Medicine*, **6**, 369–70 [DOI: 10.1038/74610]

Noble, M. (2000b) 'Can neural stem cells be used to track down and destroy migratory brain tumor cells while also providing a means of repairing tumor-associated damage?', *Proceedings of the National Academy of Science USA*, **97**, 12393–5 [DOI: 10.1073/pnas.97.23.12393]

Odorico, J.S., **Kaufmann, D.S.**, and **Thomson, J.A.** (2001) 'Multilineage differentiation from human embryonic stem cell lines', *Stem Cells*, **19**, 193–204 [PubMed: 11359944] [DOI: 10.1634/stemcells.19-3-193]

Pesce, M., and **Schöler, H.R.** (2000) 'Oct-4: Control of totipotency and germline determination', *Molecular Reproduction and Development*, **55**, 452–7 [PubMed: 10694754] [DOI: 10.1002/%28SICI%291098-2795%28200004%2955%3A4%3C452%3A%3AAID-MRD14%3E3.0.CO%3B2-S]

Pesce, M., and **Schöler, H.R.** (2001) 'Oct-4: Gatekeeper in the beginnings of mammalian development', *Stem Cells*, **19**, 271–6 [PubMed: 11463946] [DOI: 10.1634/ stemcells.19-4-271]

Richards, M., et al. (2002) 'Human feeders support prolonged undifferentiated growth of human inner cell masses and embryonic stem cells', *Nature Biotechnology*, **20**, 933–6 [PubMed: 12161760] [DOI: 10.1038/nbt726]

Sanchez-Ramos, J.R. (2002) 'Neural cells derived from adult bone marrow and umbilical cord blood', *Journal of Neuroscience Research*, **69**, 880–93 [PubMed: 12205681] [DOI: 10.1002/jnr.10337]

Sharpless, N.E., and **Depinho, R.A.** (2002) 'P53: Good cop/bad cop', *Cell*, **110**, 9–12 [PubMed: 12150992] [DOI: 10.1016/S0092-8674%2802%2900818-8]

Spradling, A., **Drummond-Barbosa, D.**, and **Kai, T.** (2001) 'Stem cells find their niche', *Nature*, **414**, 98–104 [PubMed: 11689954] [DOI: 10.1038/35102160]

Svejstrup, J.Q. (2002) 'Transcription repair coupling factor: A very pushy enzyme', *Molecular Cell*, **9**, 1151–2 [PubMed: 12086609] [DOI: 10.1016/S1097-2765%2802%2900553-1]

Tamashiro, K.L., et al. (2002) 'Cloned mice have an obese phenotype not transmitted to their offspring', *Nature Medicine*, **8**, 262–7 [PubMed: 11875497] [DOI: 10.1038/nm0302-262]

Taniguchi, H., et al. (1996) 'Presence of hematopoietic stem cells in the adult liver', *Nature Medicine*, **2**, 198–203 [PubMed: 8574965] [DOI: 10.1038/nm0296-198]

Terada, N., et al. (2002) 'Bone marrow cells adopt the phenotype of other cells by spontaneous cell fusion', *Nature*, **416**, 542–5 [PubMed: 11932747] [DOI: 10.1038/nature730]

Theise, N.D., et al. (2000) 'Liver from bone marrow in humans', *Hepatology*, **32**, 11–16 [PubMed: 10869283] [DOI: 10.1053/jhep.2000.9124]

Thomson, J.A. et al. (1998) 'Embryonic stem cell lines derived from human blastocytes', *Science*, **282**, 1145–7 [PubMed: 9804556] [DOI: 10.1126/science.282.5391.1145]

Till, J.E., and **McCulloch, E.A.** (1961) 'A direct measurement of radiation sensitivity of normal mouse bone marrow cells', *Radiation Research*, **14**, 213–22 [PubMed: 13776896]

Tsai, R.Y., **Kittappa, R.**, and **McKay, R.D.** (2002) 'Plasticity, niches, and the use of stem cells', *Developmental Cell*, **2**, 707–12 [PubMed: 12062083] [DOI: 10.1016/S1534-5807%2802%2900195-8]

Turker, M.S. (2000) 'Somatic cell mutations: Can they provide a link between aging and cancer?', *Mechanisms of Ageing and Development*, **117**, 1–19 [PubMed: 10958919] [DOI: 10.1016/S0047-6374%2800%2900133-0]

Wakayama, T., et al. (2001) 'Differentiation of embryonic stem cell lines generated from adult somatic cells by nuclear transfer', *Science*, **292**, 740–43 [PubMed: 11326103] [DOI: 10.1126/science.1059399]

Watt, F.M., and **Hogan, B.L.** (2000) 'Out of Eden: Stem cells and their niches', *Science*, **287**, 1427–30 [PubMed: 10688781] [DOI: 10.1126/science.287.5457.1427]

Whetton, A.D., and **Graham, G.J.** (1999) 'Homing and mobilization in the stem cell niche', *Trends in Cell Biology*, **9**, 233–8 [PubMed: 10354570] [DOI: 10.1016/S0962-8924%2899%2901559-7]

Wilmut, I., et al. (1997) 'Viable offspring derived from fetal and adult mammalian cells', *Nature*, **385**, 810–13 [PubMed: 9039911] [DOI: 10.1038/385810a0]

Wobus, A.M. et al. (2002) 'Embryonic stem cells as a model to study cardiac, skeletal muscle, and vascular smooth muscle cell differentiation', *Methods in Molecular Biology*, **185**, 127–56 [PubMed: 11768985]

Woods, N.B., **Ooka, A.**, and **Karlsson, S.** (2002) 'Development of gene therapy for hematopoietic stem cells using lentiviral vectors', *Leukemia*, **16**, 563–9 [PubMed: 11960333] [DOI: 10.1038/sj.leu.2402447]

Yeom, Y.L., et al. (1996) 'Germline regulatory element of Oct-4 specific for the totipotent cycle of embryonal cells', *Development*, **122**, 881–94 [PubMed: 8631266]

Ying, Q.L., et al. (2002) 'Changing potency by spontaneous fusion', *Nature*, **416**, 545–8 [PubMed: 11932748] [DOI: 10.1038/nature729]

Yoshimizu, T., et al. (1999) 'Germline-specific expression of the Oct-4/green fluorescent protein (GFP) transgene in mice', *Development, Growth and Differentiation*, **41**, 675–84 [DOI: 10.1046/j.1440-169x.1999.00474.x]

PART II
Law

Chapter Four

Human Biotechnology, Transculturality, Globalization and Symbolic (Criminal) Law

Carlos María Romeo Casabona

1. Transculturality and Globalization

1.1. *A New Scenario for Biotechnological Law: Globalization*

By and large, the realistic and potential uses of research findings, of work with human genotypes, and of innovations that could give rise to new knowledge in the field of biotechnology are known. Specifically in the area of human biotechnology, the focus falls mainly on the two areas that have the most significance for humankind: health (diagnostic procedures and medical treatment) and reproduction, which is sometimes related to a couple's or an unborn child's health problems.

Undoubtedly, work on the methods and products of biotechnology (as well as on the research that supports it) should be consistent with the already existing precautionary and security measures for the handling of living matter. This becomes even more imperative when these procedures involve genetic engineering, because the consequences of this manipulation, both in humans and in other living things, remain unpredictable.

Of all the issues related to the complex field of human biotechnology, I shall be concentrating on those that are related directly to our basic rights, in particular to those dealing with life and physical and moral integrity, and how they are proclaimed through several international legal channels and the constitutions of a number of countries. The legal systems recognize that life and the integrity of human beings and, in a restricted sense, the unborn (that is, in vitro and in vivo embryos or foetuses) are protected under the law. Therefore, they should be more intensely protected. This is possible through criminal law.

On the other hand, human dignity, the foundation upon which human rights and basic rights are based, can be violated by new developments in biotechnology, for example via clinical trials. The question now is to find out whether legally protected (individual as well as collective) subjects, which are sufficiently relevant and at the same time so concrete that one can resort to legal means for their protection, which is always an *ultima ratio*, are derivable.

First of all, the characteristics of these actions must be defined unambiguously from the standpoint of a hypothetical use of penal law as an instrument of control for biotechnological methods that deviate from the norm. This holds not only for an assessment of whether and how the aforementioned normative intervention might transpire, but is also a question of comparative law.

The speed at which discoveries and new applications in this field are being made must be addressed. This relates not only to the dynamics and sense of competition that exists between the various research groups, but also to the public apprehension triggered by the fact that many of these discoveries put the stability of the most widespread social perceptions to the test. This apprehension also exposes the inability of the traditional legal practices alone to offer effective and/or reassuring answers.

Second, the research upon which these biotechnological innovations rely does not require an extraordinary infrastructure or material resources, which means that it is neither costly nor difficult to carry out. The decisive factor pertains to the qualification of the researcher in his respective field. This means that this work could potentially be carried out in any given country, because it is enough for a small group of researchers, supported by a minimal infrastructure and nominal resources, to come together. Furthermore, this can take place regardless of the capabilities of the researchers of the respective country.

Third, it must be emphasized that the cultural particularities, especially moral, religious and legal traditions, have an impact on the various ways in which countries legally handle this matter. When assessments of biotechnology are not made on a solid foundation of principles, which are unambiguously and axiologically defined from the onset, it often happens that public perception changes very rapidly and that public officials supply only mimetic answers.

Finally, the standardized role, which has contributed to the construction of the principle of human dignity for decades, must be addressed. Although it was created by Western culture, to a greater or lesser extent, it has been accepted by several non-Western societies. Specific to the field of biotechnology, there are now new contributions that should help stimulate this standardizing process, including a 1997 statement from UNESCO regarding the human genotype and human rights as well as the Council of Europe's Convention on Human Rights and Biomedicine (1997) and the accompanying protocols. In a certain sense, these legal measures have also contributed to a globalization of bioethics. In this respect, it is striking that a number of countries that neither have a cultural tradition in this field nor are a part of the avant-garde of biomedical research have eagerly adopted legal measures, such as patient's consent as a basic right or a hastened ban on reproductive human cloning (for example in Peru, Vietnam and the People's Republic of China, despite the fact that therapeutic cloning is permitted there).

International law had indeed supported a transcultural perspective with respect to human biotechnology, and it has probably benefited from the concurrence of a number of factors:

(1) Ethical and cultural references with regard to clear and non-controversial applications of the new biotechnologically related challenges are absent in the laws of most countries. This means that some values (human rights, right to protection under the law) that exist in connection with human biotechnology have more easily been granted universal recognition in comparison with other rights (civil, political, and rights for

certain social groups). Though the latter group emerged first, it was not always able to find counterparts in the cultural view and moral codes of other communities.

(2) The appearance and the initial development of bioethical law is by and large a 'soft law', or, in other words, a law without enforcement and serious legal consequence. Nevertheless, a number of examples tell the opposite story, particularly when human biotechnology is involved (for example, the German Embryo Protection Law).

(3) A nation's sovereignty is not compromised when international law oversees the areas of human biotechnology.

The aforementioned international legal channels have made possible not only the transcultural development of a number of bioethical principles, but also a globalizing process in the field of bioethics in the absence of transcultural integration.

1.2. The Foundations for Transcultural Law regarding Biotechnology

Efforts have been undertaken in order to establish a transcultural ethics, or rather a law that will prevent one particular dominant ethics from forcing itself upon all others. An example of this phenomenon is Western ethics, which was built upon a Christian foundation. This goal is earning increasing interest owing to the accelerated processes of economic and technological globalization and to the risks they pose to humankind. This includes also ethical and legal dimensions, particularly with regard to bioethics.

Therefore, UNESCO took the initiative to develop and adopt a 'Declaration on Universal Norms on Bioethics'.[1] This document included potentially relevant aspects of genetics and human biotechnology. It is now very important to find the foundations of a transcultural ethics, particularly when we see that other recent experiments in this field have not yielded the desired results. This is currently the case with regard to the United Nation's efforts to pass an agreement, which would ban the practices of human cloning for reproductive and so-called therapeutic purposes. The ban on reproductive cloning has found almost unanimous consensus, although we have not taken into account the fact that its illegitimacy is not clear in all cases. For example, this is true when the technology proves itself to be reliable and it is used to help an infertile couple or to prevent the transmission of a genetic disease from parent to child (Grupos de Expertos sobre Bioética y Clonación 1999: 198ff; Romeo Casabona 1997: 21ff). On the other hand, therapeutic cloning is confronted with irreconcilable cultural views regarding the respect and protection of human life in its initial stages as well as pressure from the scientific community. The problems that the Council of Europe had regarding its statement about human rights and biomedicine are also well known. Although this research does not sanction the creation of human embryos, it is permitted as long as frozen, surplus embryos are used.

We have already been warned that the task of establishing a universally accepted, transcultural ethics and law in the biotechnologies brings with it the risk that it will degenerate into a form of cultural imperialism. It is a fact of history that every society has a tendency to impose its culture and ethical principles on other societies.

1 Meeting of the International Commission for Bioethics, UNESCO, Paris, 27–29 April 2004.

It has also been pointed out that the opposite should also be avoided, namely a degeneration into particularism or communitarianism. Having said that, the rejection of a certain universality brings with it an unwanted risk of remaining in a state of relativism, in which it is not possible to identify or define universally recognized values and principles.

Among the various hypotheses upon which transcultural ethics and law should be founded (Vallespin 2004: 111ff), I now want to highlight only those which claim that an acceptable transcultural ethics must always emanate from general elements or a common ethical denominator pertinent to all the diverse cultures on this planet.

Some authors wanted to see this nominal collective point in the principle of reciprocity. According to Peter Singer, the principle of reciprocity should in effect represent the 'Golden Rule', which has been adapted in every culture and religion throughout time (Singer 2003: 154f). However, this principle has found recognition or respect neither in history (for example, in the teachings of Jesus Christ, who preached that we should love our enemies and who called upon us to turn the other cheek) nor in several of the current fundamentalist factions (for example, in the radical movements, which Singer himself observed). Although this principle still attracts attention, it appears inadequate as the 'glue' of a universal ethics. This is certainly still of interest today in view of the cultural achievements of our civilization, which share particular characteristics.

That said, the theory of human rights has a deep-rooted ethical background and an undeniable value relative to its universal acceptance. This is also in view of international recognition, which human rights gained by international legislation and upon which some of these rights enjoy indisputable universality. The concept developed on the basis of human rights has a downside: it presents the overemphasis of the individual typical of western culture, which is contrary to a collectivist worldview present in other cultures (for example, in the Far East; some parts of Africa; and the indigenous peoples of the Americas). Supported by a holistic standpoint, the latter view bases itself on the fact that when the community takes responsibility for its members and vice versa, it is possible to bring about harmony in the community. Through this, the community will earn the respect of its members.

Without having to delve into such a seductive debate, it is clear that either way one should take advantage of the universal recognition that to human rights have and that this should be used as a reference point in order to identify and embrace all common ethical and judicial values and to collectively share them. What is more, human rights are neither static nor do they serve to create a self-contained universe. Instead, they are in a state of perpetual evolution, in which new laws are incorporated in accordance with the needs of humanity. For this reason, they are a very valuable instrument in the shaping of new laws in the domains of genetics and biotechnology.

Specifically pertaining to the above-mentioned domains and biomedicine in general, is what we find in the statement from UNESCO and in the work and legal resources of the Council of Europe, namely the crux of common and shared values that have been concretized in new and renewed human rights. A commendable swing in the direction of a more collectivist view of human rights can be discerned in statements from UNESCO, concerning the protection of the interests of future generations (statement about the responsibility of current generations towards future generations, 1997) and solidarity between nations (universal statement about the human genotype and human rights, 1997).

Consequently, the present challenge is to ensure that ethical globalization takes place within a transcultural framework. Within this framework, universal recognition for certain shared values and laws will be accepted, which, in turn, can provide us with answers to challenges facing a globalized world. Unfortunately, these points can only be listed in this article. In order to continue moving in this direction, it is necessary to recognize how individual factors can be merged with collective principles and rights. This should then serve as the axiological framework, also with regard to co-existence, that needs to be both created and strengthened in the coming decades.

As the list would be endless, I shall limit it by mentioning only those aspects that I believe to be indispensable to the scope of globalization.

I consider the principles of responsibility (Jonas 1984), solidarity, justice (Rawls), equality, tolerance (Kaufmann 1999), non-discrimination, and responsibility for future generations (Romeo Casabona 2002) to be the indispensable foundation of our civilization. These principles or rights have an additional importance because they have both individual and collective dimensions. In this article, I shall not delve into the contents of any of these principles for one of two reasons: because they are already well known or because they are so complex that they would merit a monographic study.

Despite their importance, we must be aware that they are not rights or principles embraced by all cultures, and even in the West they have hardly been adopted, or at least not as legal norms. A demand for a balance and counterbalance against the serious risks becomes even more critical because globalization is perpetually spreading and intensifying. Moreover, these risks radiate from several power sources that cannot be controlled by nations or the international community with our current resources. At the moment, the field of biotechnology presents us with the attractive temptation to cross all boundaries and to evade all means of control. Human rights could serve as an appropriate instrument, which, as a first step, could limit this.

I would now like to reflect briefly on the principle of human rights and human dignity (Romeo Casabona 1994: 44ff, 67ff). There is no doubt about its Western origins. Regardless of this, it can offer a collective perspective (in connection with the dignity of a people), and human dignity represents a protagonistic paradigm of an individual's utmost significance within society. Undoubtedly, this has earned recognition as a more or less universal principle, although it is generally not described as a 'basic right'.[2] Instead, it is a human characteristic that is legally projected onto our basic rights. The importance of human dignity as a boundary and barrier against potential misuses of human biotechnology is unparalleled (Cortina 2004: 29) because it bans the use of humans, meaning in all stages of development, solely as a means to an end. By using it as a voice of authority, the term 'human dignity' has unfortunately been overused and misappropriated in connection with a

2 Cf. the German Constitution, which states that human dignity is a basic right (Art. 1), at least according to the majority opinion.

number of advances in biomedical science. As a result, we have evaded a dialogue and the possibility to reach common ground and consensus. Nevertheless, I am of the opinion that the notion and significance of human dignity need to be reinforced because its contribution to the field of human biotechnology is only valuable when it is used judiciously and sincerely.

There are cases of intention to select certain biological traits that are considered to be desirable, for example through pre-implantation diagnosis and pre-implantation genetic diagnosis. There are other cases that imply genetic engineering. However, I ask myself whether this definition of human dignity is sufficient to deal with the various situations associated with this group of cases; that is, genetic engineering. Genetic engineering implies conflicts that exist beyond the individual dimension, because there is a collective dimension involved. The human race as a whole could be affected.

We have yet to consider whether human dignity might not also have a supra-individualist dimension in such situations. Some forthcoming uses of genetic engineering as a means of optimization (that is, which could be considered a form of eugenics, if carried out using gametes before reproduction or in the zygote) could have the potential to affect all human beings or particular ethnic groups in that the genetic design that sets them apart from other species or ethnicities could be modified. Consequently, future generations would be affected. Aside from specific individuals who could be affected, a different definition of human dignity, applied supra-individually, could help prevent these types of practices. Maybe it could offer us also an unambiguous standpoint with regard to defining 'normal' and 'pathological'. On the other hand, globalization processes almost certainly necessitate this same consideration in questions of human dignity. For this reason, we need to keep in mind UNESCO's statement about 'the responsibility of current generations towards future generations'.[3] It declares that 'the human genome should be protected with complete respect in relation to human dignity and human rights. Advances in science and technology cannot in any way endanger the preservation of either humankind or of any other species' (Art. 6).

2. The Function of Criminal Law in the face of New Biotechnological Dangers

It has been brought into question whether the functionality of criminal law in particular and the efficiency of law in general can combat unwanted practices that have roots in the biotechnological domain. This train of thought must be presented within a larger context, in which a legitimate use of criminal law is discussed with regard to new dangers and risks, which are tied to more complex social activities (Hassemer 1992: 378ff, and 2000: 271; Herzog 1991: 21ff; Prittwitz 1993: 17ff).[4] This includes economic and financial activities protected by underground criminal organizations, in which it is impossible to determine exactly who is responsible; industrial and biotechnological activities that apparently pose unforeseeable risks

3 Statement from UNESCO, 11 December 1997.

4 See also papers published by the Institute for Criminal Science in Frankfurt, 2000.

to life, our wellbeing and the environment; the spread of new information and communication technology, and so on.

As a result, one has the impression that it is not easy to determine who or what are legal assets, particularly when they have a collective character, meaning that they are 'diffused'. One also has the feeling that we are trying to prevent practices linked with real and uncertain risks instead of dealing with violations against those people and entities protected under the law (because of this, criminal law is not related to the principle of non-maleficence); that criminal law is in fact unrelated to the actual dealings with punishment with regard to general risks, and in this sense it corresponds more with administrative law (a Spanish author describes it as a bureaucratization of criminal law; Silva Sánchez 1999: 100) in that such tasks are a part of this legal area. These circumstances have led us to reject criminal law as an appropriate means of prevention with regard to the new risks threatening our postmodern society. This line of action deprives criminal law of its preventative effectiveness. In this way, it would be given only a symbolic function and thereby would be stripped of its legitimacy (Arroyo Zapatero, Neumann & Nieto Martín 2003: 225ff).

The debate against the use of criminal law stipulates variable regulation of the activities mentioned, including those in the biotechnological domain. These are formal and informal social controls with diverse natures and judicial mechanisms that are anchored in administrative law, which would mean that only a narrow space for criminal law would remain; according to the opinions of the most substantiated positions, no space would remain.

In the following section, I shall examine briefly what influence has been exerted upon legislators by the phenomena of transculturality and globalization. I shall also investigate whether the preceding critique of the use of criminal law is acceptable in cases where we wish to prevent certain practices in the biotechnological domain through the use of judicial protection means; that is, judicial mechanisms which legal order offers or should offer. Furthermore, this will also be pursued in reference to objects and subjects protected under the law that are affected by genetic engineering and human biotechnology.

2.1. The Possibility for Criminal Law to exert a Preventative Function with regard to Human Biotechnology

An assessment of the practicability of the use of criminal law in the biotechnological domain, and, over and above that, the possibility that that type of law might fulfil an effective and preventative function, reaches beyond the difficulties relevant to the activities of a postmodern society. An example of this is related to the need for clear-cut identification of those legal assets which will be affected. The problem concerns more than a practicable description of criminal practices that are included in the facts constituting an offence or in the appropriateness of traditional criteria of responsibility now applied to these new disciplines. Biotechnology in particular faces a specific and important problem.

Numerous gene manipulations are described as theoretically or hypothetically achievable in scientific journals, although from a technical perspective they are not yet possible. At this point, the question is, do we need a preventative function now; that is, before the anticipated criminal practices can even be carried out? This fact could lead to a far-reaching criticism of the use of criminal law in this domain, because it concerns the creation of a 'future set of facts' that constitutes an offence. One should not overlook the significance of this critique, because it does indeed deal with the construction of such a set of facts including practices that are infeasible at the time that the law is passed (Romeo Casabona 1996: 431ff, and 1994: 173ff.).

Proceeding from this point, the issue now relates to the question of whether or not criminal law fulfils more a symbolic than a preventable function (Díez Ripollés 2001: 16ff). This, however, would be bound with a renunciation of its impact, which would lead to a loss of confidence in its protective powers on the part of the citizens and consequently a loss of confidence in its right even to exist. This can be seen in the following statement:

> symbolic legislation, which stigmatizes this behavior and the qualification of concrete goods, is … a clear example of a criminal code with an educational or ethical–social character. One can already see that these provisions, which have an exclusively symbolic function, cannot be legitimized and must be removed from the legal system because they lack the preventive functions that would make them legitimate (Silva Sánchez 1992: 306).

Even if the facts of the case constituting an offence can be realized, the use of criminal law against such practices has also been criticized because of its lack of enforcement. This is because it is not yet know whether these practices will in time become possible. As a result, they cannot be punishable by law, because the potential offenders are part of the scientific community and the offences will be carried out in the protected realm of the laboratory.

2.2. Preventative Criminal Law and Symbolic Criminal Law

One must take for granted that criminal law always has a symbolic content and meaning, in order to express social disapproval of certain practices, which the law calls 'offences'. This educational and social–ethical function, which is connected to the symbolic impact of criminal law, is not to be criticized.[5] On the contrary, it is an impact that has its origins in criminal evaluation standards themselves (in a positive sense with regard to legal assets; and in a negative sense in relation to the practices that threaten these subjects and objects and the practices described in the facts that constitute an offence). Nonetheless, it does not lose its primary and preventative function because it is a process that supports certain practices in order to earn respect for the legal assets. For this reason, criminal law is not so removed from its functions, which are understood primarily as protection under the law (Cerezo Mir 1996: 15; Roxin 1997: 19f).

It is true that this should not be the only or principal function of criminal law, so that legislators fulfil their duty of creating and implementing a new set of facts

---

5 With regard to this, one should keep in mind the aforementioned objections raised by Silva Sánchez (1992: 306).

constituting an offence, although legislators know that this is ineffective. The main function of criminal law is to prevent the most serious assaults on socially relevant legal assets, even when they seem to play only a minor role. For example, this is the case with dangerous abstract offences or risky offensive actions by which legal protection is *ratio legis* (Roxin 1997: 19). Hassemer thinks that the question is not whether or not criminal law has a symbolic impact, but rather at what point such impacts should be acknowledged (Hassemer 1991: 17ff.; 23f).

> According to this, criminal law is symbolic in a critical sense in that the latent functions outweigh the blatant ones: in other words, criminal law brings with it the expectations that, in addition to those described in it, it fulfils other objectives through its norms and application (Hassemer 1991: 24).

Therefore, the question is whether it is possible to create a new set of facts constituting an offence in the biotechnological domain through which criminal law could fulfil its preventative function. This, however, needs to be accomplished without having other impacts or symbolic interests outweighing it. In order to offer a suitable answer to this question, it is necessary to distinguish between two strategies. In the first place, the question has to be answered whether it is possible for criminal policy, as presented in the biotechnological domain, to fulfil its function as a legal protection. This must then be done in the sense of *lege ferenda* and through an analysis of reform proposals. One must also identify who or what are legal assets and the practices that are punishable by law. Second, the results of the previous reflections should be compared with the possible solutions. This would confirm the assumption that the scepticism with regard to the effectiveness of criminal law in the area of biotechnology is due to the inadequate efforts of legislators (the *lege lata* perspective). In this way, the aspects relevant to an acceptable form of the set of facts constituting an offence are revealed.

2.3. Solving the Problem of the Prevention Function in Criminal Law with Respect to Human Biotechnology

It is likely that the following theory evokes fundamental objections: the symbolic side of criminal law has intensified considerably with the introduction of offences associated with human biotechnology. An innovation for criminal law is the fact that there are actions which are not yet practicable in all situations and which legislators believe to be particularly significant for the future. With this in mind, Mantovani correctly points out that lawyers are not only responsible for shaping the present in rational terms, but also for planning the future. He goes on to say that the accelerated advances in biomedicine have a tendency to translate 'future possibilities' into 'future', and then 'future' turns into 'present' (Mantovani 1993: 6). Accordingly, this diagnosis is correct and it is permissible to use legal means, including criminal law, in the biomedical field. The problem now is recognizing which scientific progress justifies the intervention of criminal law.

Criminal law is not limited to extending this impact on biotechnology (Luzón-Peña 2001: 49ff). Inasmuch are practices punishable, particularly when they are acutely serious and threatening to certain legal assets. A possible realization of such practices is reasonably foreseeable. This potentiality rightly represents a requisite minimum for the legitimization of criminal law. As a result, one cannot exclude the creation of a future set of facts constituting an offence. This last supposition is consistent with the observation that criminal law has a more restricted and modest function in the biotechnological domain because of its particular nature compared to administrative law, for example (Roxin 1997: 22).

At this point, one must remember that at its 1989 Vienna Conference the International Association of Penal Law came to the conclusion that it would be advisable to introduce a specific set of facts constituting an offence concerning gene manipulation and reproductive cloning (International Association of Penal Law, 1988). At that time, the scientific community did not believe it was possible that the technology of somatic nuclear transfer (a form of cloning), which would eventually produce 'Dolly', could be used on mammals. Nevertheless, no doubt was cast on the preventative effect of penal law in connection with more traditional, rarely committed offences.

With regard to unpunished crimes, the instigators of these practices enjoy this freedom because of the ignorance on the part of the responsible authorities to expose and persecute these offences. For this reason, apparently very little is known about how scientists in these fields carry out their work and that they are constantly under pressure to be the first to publish their results. Likewise, recognition and the prospect of receiving more funding to continue their work are contingent to their findings and the ensuing publications. Even though perhaps the earliest results do not always get published (for example, the manipulation of reproductive cells, including the extraction of human embryos in vitro), it is unreasonable to think that such findings will never come to light, because they represent the most reliable evidence of successes in science.

This yields the warning expressed by criminal law that certain research or biotechnological applications should not go in certain directions or pursue certain goals. This does not mean that there should be a general criminalization of research in these fields, because it will find a suitable framework, or, more specifically, a legitimate framework, within the legal system and in particular within the normative, regulatory, non-penal guidelines.[6]

Human reproductive cloning seems to present a clear-cut example of this preventative effect because both its punitive ban and lack of social and institutional approval have led to a point at which those researchers who claim that the technology is ready for use on human beings or say that they have already had success with it must conceal their supposed findings and maintain that the crime was committed in a place with legal immunity (at present and in view of the technical difficulties experienced by human cloning, such violations fall more into the category of fraud against those who finance such projects and potential clients).

---

6 Article 20 of the Spanish Constitution and laws 35/1988 to 15/2003 were changed in this way, 'sobre técnicas de reproducción asistida, y sobre la utilización de Embriones y fetos humanos, de sus células, tejidos u órganos' ['On methods of artificial reproduction, and on the use of the cells, tissues and organs of human embryos'].

From a global perspective and taking into consideration the various facts constituting an offence in the most representative countries, one does not have the impression that they are in breach of the minimum requirement for punitive intervention; or if they are in breach, it is of little significance. They show both an ignorance of the scientific research or reality that they are supposed to be prohibiting and a lack of good law-making practice.

In this way, the principle of minimal intervention was violated in a number of cases: in Germany (the Embryo Protection Law from 1990), in Brazil (the law from 2005) or France (the law from 2004).

3. Symbolic Criminal Law and Techniques for the Typification of Criminal Practices

Even if we conclude that preventative criminal law is compatible both with the punishment of some practices associated with gene manipulation in human beings, even though they remain difficult to criminally prosecute, and with the typification of criminal practices that are not yet realizable, though they will very likely be possible in the future, the final answer with regard to the existence of such offences is dependent on the assessment of the typification systems in the wording of the law. Keeping this in mind, I would now like to address briefly the law-making techniques leading to this typification of criminal offences, which is still neglected by doctrine and legislators (Díez Ripollés 2003); Sanchez-Lazaro (in press).

Despite the difficulties that arise from the creation of new offences, legislators must act with the utmost judiciousness. The current uneasiness and interest triggered by the mere indication of certain practices in the biotechnological domain have caused legislators to react immediately in a number of cases, even though they sometimes do not know what they should make punishable. Furthermore, this occurs without their realizing and maybe also without asking themselves which interests – that is, legal assets – need to be protected. Afterwards, they are content with the fact that they have pacified the public. (This is the symbolic effect of criminal law in a narrow sense.)

The preventative effectiveness of an offence, its criminal and political justification and possible critique, because of its purely symbolic effect, are ultimately hinged upon a fulfilment of certain typification requirements of legislative techniques.

For this reason, legislators should consider the following principles, which I shall now briefly describe.

(1) The identification or creation of a legal asset deserving of protection by criminal law. First of all, a legal asset or assets should be clearly identified. At the same time, it is necessary to define the ownership of these individual or supra-individual legal assets. By defining the legal assets, several offences are also identified, which protect the same legal asset (or something very similar) and include concurrently the systematic location of new offences that share with the others either identity or similarity of legal assets. Additionally, in cases in which it is not possible to find this kind of relationship,

we can use the ownership of legal assets as a supplementary criterion in the search for a legal stance.[7]

(2) Demarcation of the materiality of an action. The materiality of an action must also be defined in order to arrive at a better concretization of the various modalities of action that can point to the action that is being typified.

(3) The selection of practices worthy of punishment. It is equally important that practices that may pose a greater risk of injury to these legal assets have priority in the selection of potentially criminal practices. Conversely, it is necessary to guard against the danger that the description of elements of an offence and their modality are too closely bound to a specific procedure, which at the same time excludes other modalities that could be developed in the future. In fact, this proves to be true in some cases in which certain technical innovations bring into question the validity of the description of objective elements that constitute an offence. One such example concerns the creation of embryos using nuclear transfer, but without the goal of reproduction. (If this were the case, then this practice could fall into the category of offences relating to human cloning.)

(4) The selection of the structure of facts that constitute an offence. The next step is defined by the choice of a suitable technique for typifying criminal offences that are to be prevented. Furthermore, this is to be done on the level of a more or less preset criminal intervention. An analysis of this leads legislators to make the following decision: whether the elements constituting an offence are developed as an offence resulting in injury or endangerment (successful offence) or, in contrast, as a simple or single offence that is not dependent on its success or failure (an abstract endangerment or dangerous offence).

    The subjective component of the structure of elements constituting an offence is to be decided over and above the punishment of negligent practices that are only penalized as an exception.

(5) An exact description of actions that constitute an offence. The already constructed elements of a case that constitute an offence must be comprehensible for potential norm recipients: both prohibited and desired practices need to be explicitly articulated.

    Right now, this lack of clarity regarding criminal offences in the biotechnological domain is remarkable.

(6) Illegality. Cases that are in fact permitted by law should be clearly described in the wording of the law. In the biotechnological domain, it is possible that no framework for permissibility for practices that constitute an offence remains; consequently, the fact that a practice constitutes an offence already implies that it is illegal.

(7) The legal consequences: comparability and suitability. Legislators must also carefully assess aspects such as punishment, possible security measures, or even minor consequences.

(8) Sub-law or criminal code. Along with the already mentioned decisions, legislators must make one more, which will eventually become the most important even though it is logically hinged on the previous selections. More specifically, it concerns the

7 In the Spanish Criminal Code from 1995, one can find a flawed classification of offences under the same heading that describes the various legal assets.

decision to introduce the new facts of the case constituting an offence either into the criminal code or as a special law.

4. Summary

International law has supported a transcultural perspective in connection with human biotechnology. This transcultural perspective has probably garnered support through the fact that in the realm of national law, ethical and cultural references, whose applicability is unambiguous and indisputable are missing with respect to the new challenges presented by human biotechnology. In connection with this, contributions in this direction, such as UNESCO's universal statement about the human genotype and human rights (1997) and the Council of Europe's agreement about human rights and biomedicine (1997) should be acknowledged.

However, in the domains of human genetics and biotechnology we find also an undesirable (though sometimes unavoidable) 'soft law' and a number of 'soft values', which can give rise to the following:

(1) Contradictory values in national legislation. This occurs when the legislative framework for research concerning the protection of human test tube embryos promotes on the one hand a fierce protection of test tube embryos, but also, on the other hand, the practices that render them vulnerable.
(2) A perspective of globalization which is not transcultural, such as an absolute ban of the practice of human cloning within those countries that passed legislation against it; or hiding behind some form of symbolic justice, where law-makers show more concern for the moral and social denial of certain activities and the pacification of society than for a just and effective outcome for the legal situation (although this is likely to happen in the future).
(3) Resorting to a symbolic law which is housed within a framework that appears to be concerned more with the moral and social disapproval of certain activities and the pacification of the public than with effective legal prosecution (because some activities will only emerge in the future). The problem lies not in the inefficiency of law (and punishment) to create an effective preventive defence role for protected interests, but rather in the failure of the authorities responsible for providing appropriate law-making strategies.

Bibliography

Arroyo Zapatero, L., Neumann, U., and Nieto Martín, A. (eds) (2003) *Crítica y justificación del derecho penal en el cambio de siglo*, La Mancha, Cuenca: Ediciones de la Universidad Castilla

Cerezo Mir, J. (1996) *Curso de Derecho Penal Español* – Parte General I., fifth edn, Madrid: Ed. Tecnos

Cortina, A. (2004) 'Una ética transnacional de la corresponsabilidad', in V. Serrano (ed.), *Ética y Globalización*, Madrid: *Biblioteca* Nueva

Díez Ripollés, J.L. (2001) 'El derecho penal simbólico y los efectos de la peña', in: *Actualidad Penal*, 1, **16**ff.

Díez Ripollés, J.L. (2003) *La Racionalidad de las Leyes Pénales*, Madrid: Trotta

Eser, A. (1998) 'La clonación humana Fundamentos biológicos y valoración ético-jurídica', *Revista de Derecho y Genoma Humano/Law and the Human Genome Review*, 9, 91ff.

Grupo de Expertos sobre Bioética y Clonación. (1999) *Informe sobre la clonación y Fundación Ciencias de la Salud*, Madrid: Ed. Siete Calles

Hassemer, W. (1991) 'Derecho penal simbólico y protección de bienes jurídicos', *Nuevo Foro Penal*, 51, 17ff. (23f.)

Hassemer, W. (1992) 'Kennzeichen und Krisen des modernen Strafrechts', in *Zeitschrift für Rechtspolitik*, 378ff.

Hassemer, W. (2000) 'Perspektiven einer neuen Kriminalpolitik', in his *Strafen im Rechtsstaat*, Baden-Baden: Nomos, 271ff.

Herzog, F. (1991) *Gesellschaftliche Unsicherheit und strafrechtliche Daseinsvorsorge – Studien zur Vorverlegung des Strafrechtsschutzes in den Gefährdungsbereich*, Schenck, Heidelberg: *Decker's Verlag*

International Association of Penal Law (1988) 'Droit pénal et techniques biomédicales modèrnes', *Revue de Droit Pénal et de Criminologie*, **59**, 550–1371

Jonas, H. (1984) *Das Prinzip Verantwortung, Versuch einer Ethik für die technologische Zivilisation*, Frankfurt am Main: Suhrkamp

Kaufmann, A. (1999) *Filosofía del Derecho*, Santa Fé de Bogotá: Universidad Externado de Columbia

Kriminalwissenschaftliches Institut Frankfurt (eds) (2000) *La Insostenible Situación del Derecho Penal,* Granada: Ed. Comares

Luzón-Peña, D.M. (2001) 'Función simbólica del derecho penal y delitos relativos a la manipulación genética, in C.M. Romeo Casabona (ed.), *Genética y Derecho Penal*, Bilbao et al.: Cátedra Interuniversitaria de Derecho y Genoma Humano Fundación BBVA – Diputación Foral de Bizkaia y Editorial Comares, 49ff.

Mantovani, F. (1993) 'Manipolazioni Genetiche', *Digesto Pénale, 8, 40*

Prittwitz, C. (1993) *Strafrecht und Risiko – Untersuchungen zur Krise von Strafrecht und Kriminalpolitik in der Risikogesellschaft*, Frankfurt am Main: Klostermann

Romeo Casabona, C.M. (1994) 'Legal limits on human experimentation', in BBV Foundation (ed.), *The Human Genome Project: Legal Aspects*, Madrid: BBV Foundation, 173ff.

Romeo Casabona, C.M. (1994) *El Derecho y la Bioética ante los límites de la vida humana*, Madrid: Ed. Centro de Estudios Ramón Areces

Romeo Casabona, C.M. (1996) *Del Gen al derecho*, Santa Fé de Bogotá: Serv. Publicaciones Universidad Externado de Colombia

Romeo Casabona, C.M. (1997) 'Legal limits on research and its results? The cloning paradigm', *Revista de Derecho y Genoma Humano / Law and the Human Genome Review*, 6, 21ff.

Romeo Casabona, C.M. (2001) Aportaciones del principio de precaución al derecho penal, in *Modernas Tendencias en la Ciencia del Derecho Penal y en la Criminología*, Madrid: Universidad Nacional de Educación a Distancia, 77ff.

Romeo Casabona, C.M. (2002) *Los genes y sus leyes – El derecho ante el genoma humano*, Bilbao et al.: Cátedra Interuniversitaria Fundación BBVA – Diputación Foral de Bizkaia de Derecho y Genoma Humano y Editorial Comares

Romeo Casabona, C.M. (ed.) (2004) *El principio de precaución*, Bilbao et al.: Cátedra Interuniversitaria Fundación BBVA – Diputación Foral de Bizkaia de Derecho y Genoma Humano y Editorial Comares

Roxin, C. (1997) *Strafrecht – Allgemeiner Teil – Grundlagen – Der Aufbau der Verbrechenslehre*, third edn, München: Beck

Sánchez-Lázaro, F. (in press) *¿Cómo se élabora una propuesta de lege ferenda? – Reflexiones sobre la formulación de los preceptos jurídico-pénales*, first part, Tipicidad

Silva Sánchez, J.M. (1992) *Aproximación al Derecho Penal contemporáneo*, Barcelona: Bosch

Silva Sánchez, J.M. (1999) *La expansión del Derecho penal – Aspectos de la política criminal en las sociedades postindustriales*, Madrid: Civitas

Singer, P. (2003) *Un Solo Mundo y la Ética de la Globalización,* Barcelona: Piados

Vallespín, J. (2004) 'El problema de la fundamentación de una ética global', in V. Serrano (ed.), *Ética y Globalización*, Madrid: Biblioteca Nueva, 111ff.

Chapter Five

Human Biotechnology as a Legal Challenge

Jürgen Simon

1. Introduction

We rely on lawyers to 'solve' multi-faceted problems within the law without having to be experts on the topic in question and without being particularly creative.[1] They use their methods of thinking to organize reality, and each respective reality is a blueprint of the legal organization. Such a reality supplies the contents in the form of numerous case variations, according to which reality should be categorized and organized according to useability. However, the legal system faces a challenge when the normal expectations of the public go too far because the case in question is, for some reason, particularly difficult to regulate. But what are the 'normal expectations', and what are the reasons for a challenge to law?

On 26 February 2004, the German Association of Judges released a statement in which it said that the legal system in Germany:

> has brought about legal security in all areas, also for the good of the economy and for Germany as a place for financial investment. Whoever enters into a contract in Germany can be sure that a fair solution can be found in a reasonable amount of time should a conflict arise. This makes the negotiations easier, which is obvious when one considers that a contract written in Germany is maybe ten pages long, whereas in the US a contract is typically 50 to 100 pages long and requires the work of several lawyers.[2]

According to this statement, legal security, as a secularized guarantee for justice, is one of the greatest goods. The law should be rational, plausible and consistent. The public, as user of the law, expects exactly this: the control of a reality, which may be plagued by conflict, in the sense that that reality will then be secure. The law should work according to a system similar to the one that regulates traffic: we are protected when we walk over the pedestrian crossing; we are penalized when we ignore traffic signs, drive too fast or disturb the flow of traffic. Traffic has been translated into a system of symbols, which communicate with drivers (users) and vice versa. Stolleis, following Luhman, puts it this way, 'The law as a differentiated, specialized system of communication stabilizes expectations with respect to our conduct. In this way, it

---

1 This is their legal duty according to Article 19, Section 4 of the German Constitution.

2 German Association of Judges, North Rhine-Westphalia Chapter, 26 February 2004.

controls our consciousness and behaviour and thereby acts as a deterrent' (Stolleis 2003: 7).

This stabilization of behaviour expectations and deterrence through the law is valid firstly for visible dangers: for example, we must protect ourselves from dangers such as a moving car, a loose tile on the roof or a flood.

How can concerns about the 'new scientific and technical dangers' be regulated and likewise apply to the public's expectations for security (Stolleis 2003: 7)? How has it applied to such dangers that have posed challenges to law since the 1950s: nuclear risk, major chemical disasters, global warming and now gene or nano technology? Even if lawyers happen to be familiar with the subject (which is more the exception than the rule) and are experts, scientific discoveries together with the concentrated power of economic interests are typically in an advantageous position. 'The law will continue to follow behind, at least as long as lawyers, representatives and society as a whole do not grasp or discuss what it is even about' (Stolleis 2003: 7). This is all the more true on the international level of globalization and with regard to attempts to control reality by means of international law. But how can it be regulated at all?

2. Xenotransplantation as an Example of Control through Law

We will now take a look at an example from biotechnology, xenotransplantation, because here we are dealing with the control of risks that neither scientists nor lawyers are capable of assessing. It is also a question of how dealing with these risks is addressed.

Successful organ transplantation is one of the most important achievements in medicine in the last century. However, complete realization of this medical promise is barred for reasons including an ever-present organ deficit and the problem of organ rejection. On the one hand, this worldwide deficit of transplantable organs, and on the other hand, the achievements in biotechnology and immunology, have awoken the interest of scientists to take a closer look at xenotransplantation. It is a question of using living animal cells, tissues and organs in order to battle a range of diseases.

Although the possible advantages seem to be significant, the use of xenotransplantation is not without its challenges. These include the risk of transmitting infection from animals to humans, the problem of 'informed consent', and so on. Many of those involved – for example, patients and their families, doctors, scientists, the pharmaceutical industry, interest groups for human and animal rights – are stakeholders with regard to the potential use of this groundbreaking advance in medicine. Politicians and policy must take all of these people and factors, with all of their complicated interrelationships, into consideration. For years, xenotransplantation was discussed intensively in light of legal, ethical, social and economic aspects with the goal of creating an adequate instrument for regulation while at the same time undermining critical positions. However, potential risks for individuals, beneficiaries, society and animals were also taken into account. The goal of a coordination of interests converged with a statement from the European

Commission for 'Precautionary Principle' released on 2 February 2000. It reads, 'it helps to control the dilemma of balancing the freedom and right of individual, industry and organizations with the need to reduce the risk to adverse effects to the environment, human, animal and plant health [...] finding the correct balance so that the proportionate, non-discriminatory, transparent and coherent actions can be taken requiring a structured decision-making process with detailed scientific and other objective information.'[3]

How can we reach the goal of a controlled authorization of clinical trials (with an acceptable amount of risk) and the necessary follow-up care? In this case, follow-up care means 'monitoring' patients and probably also those with whom they come into contact. Moreover, precautions for protecting against infection also include prevention.

At the turn of the twenty-first century, a number of studies were written about this topic, for example from the Nuffield Council about the 'Advisory Group on Ethics of Xenotransplantation', the Swiss Science Council, the European Council, OECD, the WHO, and so on. In these studies, the security problem was named as one of the central challenges. At the same time, there is also an essential problem of the distribution of risk between individual and collective health care interests. The Swiss Science Council, for example, stresses the need for a choice between the public's right to safety and the right of a few patients to survive and still enjoy a good quality of life. The main problem of all of these studies is recognizing the danger with regard to which risks are taken by the patients, their relatives and the hospital staff, and how those involved and finally society as a whole should deal with such risks. The problem of monitoring patients and their social surroundings after surgery is discussed in the same way as questions of the possible obligatory steps that must be carried out to quarantine these patients when xenogenic infections develop, in addition to questions regarding how far the considerable changes to their social conditions should go. According to every study, monitoring may be necessary for a limited amount of time. The Swiss study (Engels et al. 1998) starts with the necessity for various measures and certain circumstances, for example:

- life-long monitoring of the patient's health and tests for pathogens;
- accompanying research programmes for finding unknown pathogens;
- quarantining of the patient if symptoms of an infection become apparent; and
- monitoring of the hospital staff's health after coming into contact with a transplantation recipient.

However, the studies do not provide overly precise answers relating to how to deal with relatives and others who come into close contact with the patient. In this case, extensive regulation is considered to be essential. However, in a study from the Netherlands, there is doubt as to whether these critical monitoring procedures are legally feasible and organizationally possible, particularly with regard to an effective involvement of a patient's social environment.

3 With regard to the tenets of the 'Precautionary Principle' and its use in environmental protection, see also Simon and Fischer 2004.

I would now like to mention two examples that embody two very different possibilities for regulation reform: on the one hand, the United Kingdom, and on the other, Germany. The Steering Group of the United Kingdom Xenotransplantation Interim Regulatory Authority, which is responsible for working on a legal blueprint for a possible law, came to the conclusion in their report that the personal freedom of an individual, contrary to the Human Rights Act of 1998, needs to be considerably restricted.[4] In Germany, however, there is no direct regulation of xenotransplantation, but rather 'only' a law regarding protection from infection,[5] which can be referred to in conflict situations.

2.1. United Kingdom

According to the report, limitations on an individual's personal freedom should apply to those people who are closely connected to transplantation recipients; that is, the 'intimate contacts'. These include members of the household, sexual partners, and all others who are in sufficiently close contact with the recipient that the exchange of bodily fluids is possible:

- Recipients should be monitored for the rest of their lives, even if the transplant was a success or if others could be put in danger.
- Samples should be taken regularly.
- Recipients must take antibodies for the rest of their lives.
- Pregnancy and paternity should be ruled out.
- Recipients should be reachable at all times.
- Recipients should make any absences known beforehand.
- Details of additional contact persons should be provided.
- Data and samples should be stored for the duration of the recipient's life.
- Every new doctor should be made aware of the recipient's status.

Even the 'intimate contacts' have to provide samples and undergo examinations and tests, and their data and samples will then be kept for an indefinite amount of time; they must also make information for research available and be reachable at any time.

According to the report, all of these measures should take place voluntarily and on the basis of 'informed consent'. However, this raises questions about practicability, violations against human dignity, the right to live one's own life, and so on. In cases of extreme infectious xenozoonosis, the Public Health Act for disease control should be compulsorily put into use. As a side note, the Public Health Act was created in 1984.

---

4 Draft report of the Infection Surveillance Steering Group of the UKXIRA, July 1999.

5 A law to reorganize epidemiological regulations.

2.2. The German Law regarding Protection from Infection

In comparison with a far-reaching system for controlling the dangers, I would now like to discuss the newer German law regarding the protection from infection that replaced the old law intended to protect us from epidemics and claims itself to be the most modern law of its kind in Europe. Admittedly, there is a very big difference between the (sometimes) exorbitant recommendations of a report and a regulation plan that is created by the legislative process. Nevertheless, this does not rule out a comparison between how jurisprudence and legal practice would like to take onunknown risks.

The German law does not refer directly to xenotransplantation, but an implicit goal certainly pertains to monitoring it and similar risks. In conjunction with the organization of an efficient notification system, the proposed modern protection against infection might not only be quicker at recognizing infectious diseases in general, but also reduce the risks associated with xenotransplantation through better prevention measures for the protection of the public. According to Paragraph 1 of the law, its purpose is to diagnose infections early and to prevent them from spreading.

The law also makes it possible to implement far-reaching measures to protect one or more persons from infection.

In contrast to the previous federal law protecting against epidemics, the duties have been restructured according to Paragraph 4, which the Robert Koch Institute (RKI) 'must develop in order to prepare for communicable diseases and also to detect and prevent the spread of diseases as early as possible'. Together with the responsible governmental authorities, the RKI has a central role in consulting the appropriate agencies about measures for the prevention and recognition of the spread of serious communicable disease as well as in creating guidelines. This can bring with it considerably better reaction to infections.

Likewise, the obligation to notify authorities has been expanded because in Paragraph 6 of the new law it states that a suspected disease, or rather a disease 'by name', is to be reported. The same is true of disease-causing agents in Paragraph 7, which must be reported if there is any direct or indirect evidence for them. Along this same line, evidence of acute infections must also be reported. Nevertheless, they are not regulated conclusively in the list, which covers 47 different points. It is expressly stated in direct reference to the potential risks of xenotransplantation: 'Pathogens that are not present here must be registered by name if their local or temporary appearance signalizes a serious threat to the public.' In this way, currently unknown viral infections are clearly included.[6] Moreover, necessary protection measures that could be taken by the appropriate authorities have been expanded. It is expressly stated that the basic rights of personal freedom (Article 2, Section 2, Clause 2 of the German Constitution), the freedom of assembly (Article 8 of the German Constitution) and the inviolability of the home (Article 13, Section 1 of the German Constitution) have to be restricted in this case.

With all of these regulations, the new law is very comprehensive, but at the same time the wording is appropriately cautious and seems to have included the

---

6 For a different opinion, see Jungeblodt 2001: 108.

possible risks of xenotransplantation, particularly after the surgery. In my opinion, a law so flexibly worded as this one is much more appropriate than a casuistry that is comprehensive and frequently surpassed by the diverse manifestations of reality.

3. A Legal Definition of Reality

What expectations of and challenges to biotechnology does the law now have to confront? One that is often mentioned is the definition of reality. It should be legally defined and organized in such a way that it is always easy to implement. Everyone knows that this is wishful thinking, for example when we consider the 12,000 regulations for environmental law alone. Nevertheless, the expectation is there. And how it should be realized in biotechnological law remains to be seen.

However, as a lawyer, I still see a good chance for this, namely through the abstention of regulation, or rather the particularly cautious structuring of legal reality. Despite a 20-year discussion, in Germany there is still no law on genetic testing and the Federal Ministry for Health has moved the date for the expected draft from Spring to Autumn of this year (2004), but it will still not be ready. We can see that despite typical rage over regulation, Germany distinguishes itself through constructive discretion with regard to the biotechnological domain. This is not always advantageous, particularly if we take a look at the (often) bemoaned Embryo Protection Law or the new, controversial Stem Cell Law, despite the fact that, after intensive debate both inside and outside of Parliament, the law has found majority support as a provisional democratic compromise (see also Taupitz 2002: 111ff; Simon 2002a: 215ff; Rosenau 2004: 135ff).

I think that at the moment we do not need regulations in some fields, because the research still has some way to go. For example, this is the case with xenotransplantation because we have well-tried instruments of legal finding on which we can rely. Therefore, it is my opinion that it is not necessary to come up with regulations regarding genetic testing for employers, because in connection with HIV laws and data protection guidelines, and so on, we already have a clear legal situation that prohibits all violations that genetic testing allows (Ravenstein & Simon 2003: 60ff). The same is true of genetic testing carried out for insurance companies before a policy is taken out (Simon 2001). In this case, there is a voluntary declaration of obligation by the insurance companies in effect until the end of 2006, which makes all legislative precipitance unnecessary. Within the framework of our discussion, I want to ignore the fact that, from the beginning of the debate, legislators have concentrated too much on the genetic testing methods and too little on the results, which can be applied like medical results (see also Simon 1993: 24). Without a fixation on the procedural methods of genetic testing on the part of jurisprudence and legislators, legal results could probably be reached, which, based on common law, would fit better within the existing legal system.

4. Embryonic Stem Cells, Pre-Implantation Diagnosis, and the Public's Expectations of Law

The challenges to law from the public seem to be insurmountable in these domains, because it is a matter of basic values and a fundamental understanding of our societal existence. The intensive public debates have illustrated this fact, which first reached lofty heights in biotechnological disputes.[7]

4.1. Embryonic Stem Cells

I would now like to address this topic in light of the following demands: for legal consistency, for the standardization of the system, and for resolution devoid of contradictions in assessment. These demands as well as the public's expectations of law are immanent and seem to pose an inimitable challenge.

First of all, all basic rights and those who are granted basic rights need to be addressed within the framework of our constitutional rights. It should be noted that the discussion up until now has concentrated primarily on embryo protection. Less energy has been spent in considering the health of current and future patients and how they could possibly be helped by research on embryos. Along these lines, we need to ask ourselves whether the government is allowed to intervene, and if the answer is yes, then what measures it can take. In other words, those who want to restrict research must be able to justify it. This is, of course, the same in every other field. 'In this sense, the "ethics of healing" is connected to constitutional law. Bans on research threaten this guaranteed protection' (Kopetzki 2002: 157ff).[8]

The subject of these considerations can be research on already existing cell lines or imported cell lines. The considerations can apply also to stem cells that have been obtained from embryos produced by means of in vitro fertilization. Finally, there can also be questions relating to totipotent cells, from which stem cells are obtained, and to the production of embryos themselves. According to the German Constitutional Court, it is clear that all of these methods 'as serious and systematic attempts to find out the truth' are protected by the freedom of research according to Article 5, Section 3 of the German Constitution (Hufen, 2002).

Within this context, legislators can then intervene if these interventions are appropriate, necessary and reasonable for the protection of other people and things safeguarded under the constitution. The reasons for legislative intervention are usually linked with protection of human dignity and an embryo's right to life according to Articles 1 and 2, Section 2 of the German Constitution. Objections to the freedom of research are usually supported by claims of a 'slippery slope'[9] or fears that a 'dam will break'. The objections that relate to potential misuse play no

7 See also a thorough analysis by Knoepffler 2000; Sauer 2001; Merkel 2002.

8 See also Hufen 2002.

9 Merkel considers the 'slippery slope' argument to be the 'most misused type of argument in social–ethical discussions over the last hundred years' (Merkel 2002: 263).

role in constitutional law, even if they weigh heavily on the individual and society as a whole.[10]

It is well known that the German Constitutional Court has not made a statement about human dignity regarding the status of the embryo before the fourteenth day after fertilization.[11] If embryos have a right to human dignity, we have to consider whether or not research is a breach of that dignity. This is certainly the case if embryos are produced merely for their stem cells. They would then be turned into objects and this violates the 'ban on instrumentalization'.

We need to decide whether human dignity is violated when stem cells are obtained from already existing embryos that will be neither implanted nor 'adopted'. This would be the case if we assume that 'their dying as such' is more consistent with the principle of human dignity and their right to life than the use of embryos for research which seeks to cure diseases and, in a broad sense, to protect human dignity. If we apply these constitutional criteria, then a ban on research with imported stem cells is difficult to justify. This is because donors can no longer be protected by a ban on stem cell research. And, as I have already said, based on a gradated protection of dignity and life no breach of human dignity is assumed by a part of the constitutional literature. Therefore, Hufen and others have come to the conclusion that even if we want to prevent 'consumer use of embryos', a regulation stipulating a cut-off date and the criminal threat to international research projects[12] are disproportionate in accordance with the new stem cell law because they are inappropriate and imbalanced (Hufen 2002).

4.2. Pre-Implantation Diagnosis (PID)

The question of whether or not PID is constitutionally permissible can be answered in accordance with traditional constitutional principles without breaking the legal rules of argumentation.

In this way, the basic right in Article 6 of the German Constitution, which safeguards marriage and families as well as parents' desires to have children, protects us. Clinically induced in vitro fertilization is also included. There is agreement in the fact that the basic right to life and health as well as the mother's human dignity demands that these rights should be protected (inasmuch as possible) from physical and psychological dangers during pregnancy and labour. Women are granted the right to make the final decision regarding whether or not an in vitro embryo should be implanted (Hufen 2002). Moreover, one of the most important aspects of this process is a woman's 'right to be informed'.

If legislators ban diagnostic and therapeutic procedures that could reduce the risks to the mother, then this could be seen as a breach of the above-mentioned basic right (Kopetzski 2003: 55). This is the case particularly in other countries like

10 For a differentiated argument, see Maio 2002: 162.

11 See also BVerfGE 39, 1 (41); 88, 203 (251). For a detailed discussion, see also Simon 2000b:.44ff; Taupitz 2002: 47.

12 See Romeo-Casabona 2001 for more information about international regulations; see also Friele 2001 and Taupitz 2003.

Belgium, Denmark, France, Great Britain, Italy, Norway and the US, where more than 1600 children were born after PID between January 1999 and May 2001 (Sauter 2004: 27).

In order to be able to justify a ban, an embryo at a very early stage of development (the point at which PID is carried out) has to be granted the right to human dignity. However, the infringement of rights has to be more significant than the health and dignity of the mother.

If one shares in this constitutionally based opinion, it is not easy to recognize an infringement of human dignity in the phases discussed in this article: (1) the production of an embryo to bring about a pregnancy; (2) testing for serious genetic defects; (3) the possibility to decide against implantation. If we believe that those involved are responsible for their actions and compare PID with other medical examinations, it is a matter of examining the implantability and survivability of the embryos. This kind of examination can minimize the risks in critical situations, particularly when the lives of the mother and the embryo are in danger. In such cases, this procedure can be considered medically necessary (Sauter 2004: 27). Furthermore, an examination of the embryo in the mother's womb that could lead to a medically induced abortion is inappropriate, and one could hardly expect a mother to allow this. For this reason, this aspect of the debate has been crucial in recent years. This point of view, in conjunction with its concordance with constitutional principles, can actually claim to choose the more moderate approach.

In particular, this would be valid if PID were restricted to a few approved and monitored institutes and used only in serious, medically grounded cases for abortion. It is argued that misuse could be prevented by selecting existing medical grounds for abortion in advanced pregnancies.

Regardless of the solution we consider to be the best, challenges to the law are particularly demanding because they touch on the foundations of our self-conception. Even if lawyers are able to provide plausible solutions by the use of time-honoured criteria, we need to increasingly check back with other disciplines, in the sense of a real learning process, in order to do justice to the developments in biotechnology in a social process. The public's fears, which the German Constitutional Court addressed in its 1983 ruling on a national census that insisted that these fears be taken seriously, play a role and only with determination can a law be created that successfully clarifies a legal situation.

5. Conclusion

It seems possible to create a system in which control is flexible, even if the risks that need to be monitored are unknown. As shown by the reflections on xenotransplantation, this kind of flexibility can help to reduce the complexity of the situation. In other cases, analogies to long-established legal domains can be used to find solutions. Even so-called 'soft laws', as seen in the guidelines for German MDs, are an outstanding problem-solving tool, because in this case legislators are not directly involved. Instead, it is left to those affected as the 'cheapest' and 'nearest cost avoider' (as formulated in an economic analysis of the law) to settle their affairs themselves and also be able to alter their decisions if necessary.

If the public's expectations of law and the legal system are sometimes reminiscent of secularized expectations of salvation, then we must ask whether lawyers should not be able to make use of specialized training that puts them in a position to assess the contents of biotechnology. In Germany, lawyers are not trained with this in mind. This also used to be the case in the field of environmental law. On the contrary, lawyers who researched and taught this 'far-out' area were viewed with suspicion because they were so far removed from the traditional university curriculum. 'We cannot use this to build a country!' Even when the renowned American EINSHAC Institute in Washington, which has advised presidents and has given itself the task of bringing judges and scientists together in order to solve cases, even when this Institute invites the German Constitutional Court to participate, these invitations typically go unanswered. This is not because of ignorance, but rather because this kind of 'training' is unbefitting and still not well known in Germany. However, knowledge is an essential factor in creating legal security and monitoring unknown dangers.

Bibliography

Beckmann, J.P. (2000) *Xenotransplantation von Zellen, Geweben oder Organen – Wissenschaftliche Entwicklungen und Ethisch–Rechtliche Implikationen,* Berlin et al.: Springer

Engels, E.-M., Hüsing, B., Frick, T., Menrad, K., and Reiß, T. (eds) (1998) 'Technikfolgenabschätzung Xenotransplantation', *Schweizer Wissenschaftsrat TA*, **30**, Bern

Friele, M.B. (ed.) (2001) *Embryo Experimentation in Europe: Bio-medical, legal, and philosophical aspects, Bath Neuenahr Ahrweiler:* Europäische Akademie zur Erforschung von Folgen Wissenschaftlich-Technischer Entwicklungen

Gezondheitsraad (1998) *Commissie Xenotransplantie*, in *Xenotransplantie Nr*, 01, Rijswijk

Hufen, F. (2002) '*Grundrechte für den menschlichen embryo? Ein Beitrag zur Debatte über Embryonale Stammzellen und die Präimplantationsdiagnostik' – Thesen zur Tagung, 'Welche Folgen hat die Biomedizinische Forschung?'* , 1–3 November 2002, Iserlohn

Jungeblodt, S. (2001) 'Rechtliche Aspekte der Xenotransplantation', in M. Quante and A. Vieth (eds), *Xenotransplantation – Ethische und rechtliche Probleme*, Paderborn: *Mentis, 67ff.*

Knoepffler, N. (2000) 'Menschliche *Embryonen und Medizinethische Konfliktfälle',* in Knoepffler and A. Haniel (eds), *Menschenwürde und Medizinethische Konfliktfälle,* Stuttgart et al.: Hirzel, 55ff.

Kollek, R., and Held, K. (1997) *Voraussetzungen und Implikationen der Präimplantationsdiagnostik*, Hamburg: ohne Verlag

Kopetzki, C. (2002) 'Embryonale Stammzellen im Rechtsstaat – Thesen zur künftigen "Biopolitik"', in J.W. Pichler (ed.), *Embryonalstammzelltherapie versus 'Alternative' Stammzelltherapien, Wien: Verlag Österreich, 152–72*

Kopetzki, C. (2003) 'Rechtliche Aspekte des Embryonenschutzes', in Kopetzki and U.H.J. Körtner (ed.), *Embryonenschutz – Hemmschuh für die Biomedizin?*, Wien: Manz, 49–72

Maio, G. (2001) 'Die Präimplantationsdiagnostik als Streitpunkt – Welche Argumente sind tauglich und welche nicht?', *Deutsche medizinische Wochenschrift*, **126**, 889–95 [DOI: 10.1055/s-2001-16313]

Maio, G. (2002) 'Welchen Respekt schulden wir dem Embryo? Die embryonale Stammzellforschung in medizinethischer Perspektive', *Deutsche medizinische Wochenschrift*, **127**, 160–63 [PubMed: 11807661] [DOI: 10.1055/s-2002-19698]

Merkel, R. (2002) *Forschungsobjekt Embryo – Verfassungsrechtliche und ethische Grundlagen der Forschung an menschlichen embryonalen Stammzellen*, München: Deutscher Taschenbuch-Verlag.

Ravenstein, C., and **Simon, J.** (2003) 'Top Jobs für Top Gene?', in B. Sokol (ed.), *Der gläserne Mensch – DNA-Analysen. Eine Herausforderung an den Datenschutz,* Düsseldorf: ohne Verlag, 60–80

Romeo Casabona, C.M. (2001) '*Embryonic Stem Cell Research and Therapy at European Level: Is a Common Legal Framework Needed?*', *Revista de Derecho y Genoma Humano/Law and the Human Genome Review*, 15, 121–38

Rosenau, H. (2004) 'Der Streit um das Klonen und das deutsche Stammzellgesetz', in H.-L. Schreiber (ed.), *Recht und Ethik im Zeitalter der Gentechnik – Deutsche und japanische Beiträge zu Biorecht und Bioethik, Göttingen: Vandenhoeck & Ruprecht, 135ff.*

Sauer, G.W. (2001) 'Zur rechtspolitischen und bio-ethischen Zulässigkeit von Präimplantationsdiagnostik und Embryonenforschung – Versuch über das Ganze', *Loccumer Protokolle*, **24**

Sauter, A. (2004) Präimplantationsdiagnostik – Ausnahmefall oder Routinecheck?', *Tab-Brief Nr*, **26** (June), 25–8

Simon, J. (1993) Risikoregulierung und Rechtspolitik im Bereich der Genomanalyse, in R. Damm and D. Hart (eds), *Rechtliche Regulierung von Gesundheitsrisiken*, Baden-Baden: *Nomos Verlags-Gesellschaft, 19–37*

Simon, J. (2000) 'Xenotransplantation – Regelung und Regelungsbedarf', in H. Grimm (ed.), *Xenotransplantation – Grundlagen, Chancen, Risiken, Stuttgart et al.: Schattauer, 324–9*

Simon, J. (2001) *Gendiagnostik und Versicherung – Die internationale Lage im Vergleich*, Baden-Baden: Nomos Verlags-Gesellschaft

Simon, J. (2002a) '*La ley de células troncales alemana: contenido y crítica', Revista de Derecho y Genoma Human [Law and the Human Genome Review],* 17, 215–20

Simon, J. (2002b) 'Scientific Process, Judge-Made Law and Procedural Law', in *Politeia. Rivista di etica e scelte pubbliche Nr. 65 (Le questioni bioetiche davanti alle corti: le regole sono poste dai giudici?, a cura di Amedeo Santosuosso/ Giuseppe Gennari)*, 44–50

Simon, J. (2003) 'Xenotransplantation – Regelung und Regelungsbedarf', in H. Grimm (ed.), *Xenotransplantation – Grundlagen, Chancen, Risiken, Stuttgart et al.: Schattauer, 324–9*

Simon, J., and **Fischer, C.** (2004) 'Principio de Precaucio y responsabilidad de las autoridades y functionarios – El ejemplo alemán de su implementación en la legislación medioambiental', in C.M. Romeo Casabona (ed.), *El principio de precaución, Bilbao et al.: Cátedra Interuniversitaria Fundación BBVA – Diputación Foral de Bizkaia de Derecho y Genoma Humano y Editorial Comares, 265–76*

Stolleis, M. (2003) 'Erwartungen an das Recht', *Frankfurter Allgemeine Zeitung*, **30** (*Dezember)*, 7

Taupitz, J. (2001) 'Der rechtliche Rahmen des Klonens zu therapeutischen Zwecken', *NJW*, **47**, 3433–40

Taupitz, J. (2002) 'Import embryonaler Stammzellen. Konsequenzen des Bundestagsbeschlusses vom 31.01.2001', *ZRP*, **3**, 111–15

Taupitz, J. (2003) *Rechtliche Regelung der Embryonenforschung im internationalen Vergleich*, Berlin et al.: Springer Publishing

PART III
The Church

Chapter Six

Human Biotechnology as a Social Challenge: An Inquiry into Ethical Opinion-building from a Protestant Perspective

Christoph Kähler

1. Four Opening Remarks

I was invited to this conference although I am neither a doctor nor a biologist. This means that I understand as much about the research of my colleagues here as the average college student. This raises the questions, what right do Church leaders have to get involved in the bioethical debate and to influence decisions concerning research policy, and, what is their ultimate objective?

Nevertheless, I share my limited knowledge about this topic with many of my fellow citizens, to whom medical and biological specialists are accountable: this includes non-experts such as politicians who write research policy, entrepreneurs and journalists, all of whom experts try to win over for their research interests. Also part of this group are scientists who, as a part of the academic self-governing system, regularly make decisions about research and doctrine in disciplines completely outside their area of expertise.

I am now taking on the role of what some might call 'advocate of the people'. Therefore, I am obliged to gather and discuss questions that relate to work with new scientific discoveries, though particularly in the controversial biotechnological domain. I shall then evaluate these in light of the question, how do we want to live our lives?

My questions originate from a commitment to the basic assumptions of Christian faith, which I shall willingly disclose. In my opinion, the converse is also true for those who do not share these assumptions, because in my opinion they need to articulate the reasons behind their differing worldviews. However, being here in eastern Germany, though not only here, I often miss these frank declarations of opinion and their accompanying intellectual honesty because the fact is, decisions regarding research policy correspond with deep-seated convictions. Furthermore, we are also doing the opposition justice when we attempt to understand the various levels on which it operates.[1]

---

1 The legitimacy of such questions stems not only from theological dogma, but also from what we have experienced in the last 150 years with regard to scientific discoveries and

Nonetheless, there is not just *one* Protestant view, which I could then present as a closed position *ex cathedra*. Instead, various points of view are represented not only within the scope of academically grounded Protestant ethics, but also in related statements by Church leaders. However, opinions of Church leaders tend to be of a more restrictive nature,[2] while many in the former group recommend a cautious openness. There are several reasons for this.

On the one hand, the Christian faith and a critical self-examination of it – that is, theology – developed nearly simultaneously. Even Paul wrote, 'I speak as to wise men, judge ye what I say' (1 Cor. 10:15). With this example, we can see how a Church leader's statements are subject to scrutiny by the congregation and its members. This also includes internal church-related disputes.[3] This can occur when we have the goal, 'Prove all things, hold fast that which is good' (1 Thess. 5:21).

On the other hand, the teachings of the Protestant Church are not hierarchically structured. Contrary to what many claim, this implies neither a principle of 'anything goes' nor one of complete individualization; rather, it necessitates a principle of communication. This means that the congregation (and in this case, the community) needs to seek and hopefully find a general consensus on important issues. In this respect, the freedom and personal opinion of one Christian is not enough; instead, a type of institutionalized communication among many Christians is required. This is the position that I endorse. However, we also want to encourage a similar discussion and consensus-building process within the general public pertaining to questions that affect society. The Protestant Church of Germany (PCG)'s Chamber for Public Responsibility is one such channel for communication.

Finally, ethical consequences stemming from the foundations of Christian belief are typically dependent on matters of opinion, (possibly) erroneous considerations, and decisions on matters of conscience. In most cases, they are not issues concerning orthodoxy, meaning generally accepted statements about Christian doctrine. Only

---

their socio-political interpretation and use. I am especially keeping in mind the prognoses and assessments that the respective specialists in the various domains of the natural sciences use to promote their specific field. However, these projections have never succeeded in providing a picture of what would actually happen in the future. The energy–policy debate concerning the future use of atomic energy that transpired during the second half of the last century is a good example of this phenomenon. If I see it correctly, then I would say that we are now repeating some of the patterns of debates that were already formulated at the end of the nineteenth and beginning of the twentieth century in light of discussions about discoveries in biology and their anthro-biological use. Ernst Haeckel of Jena, Germany is just one of many instructive examples.

2 The protection of human embryos can in no way be restricted. Statement from the Council of the Protestant Church in Germany regarding the current bioethical debate issued on 22 May 2001; Huber, 2002a; an overview with appendix and references to other positions from Knüppel 2001: 38–88. Körtner & Büchner argue in a different way, 2002: 27-31 (restricted to PID), and 31–4 (with regard to embryonic stem cell research (which is possible under certain conditions, 33).

3 It is agreed that here in this context the voice of the Chairman of the PCG is not more valid than that of Margot von Renesse or Klaus Tanner; instead, only the better, more plausible argument is valid.

rarely do ethical judgements develop as a direct and undeniable result of fundamental Christian ideas. However, the issue we are presently debating touches directly on the biblical notion of personhood and thereby also the central questions of Christian faith.

The fact that a general consensus within the Protestant Church is out of reach at the moment led the Chamber for Public Responsibility to publish an article in 2002 with the title, 'Treating Life with the Spirit of Love' (PCG 2002). It describes the various opinions held by Protestant theologians, particularly with regard to the right to protection granted to in vitro fertilized ova not yet implanted in the uterus, the use of so-called surplus embryos, and pre-implantation diagnosis (PID). Those who are looking for straightforward advice or even guidelines for how we should proceed will not necessarily find them here. At the least, however, this article manages to accomplish many things, namely to explain earnestly and precisely both positions and their arguments, to spare them from (sometimes) obvious polemics, and to bring together counterarguments that are typically ignored.

In some respects, this article tries to summarize this debate, at least as far as I could take note of it. Additionally, I would like to put together a catalogue of questions that need to be answered if serious and (virtually) irrevocable decisions about human biotechnology are going to be made (or legally allowed) through political means. In my opinion, we must consider complex ethical problems, shed light on the pre-conditions, and take into account the various consequences *before* these decisions are made.

2. Basis for Argumentation

2.1 The axiom that 'human beings are God's creation' is at the heart of every Christian's concept of 'human being'. The identification of the greatness, finiteness and limitations of every human being follows from this axiom. Man's greatness, and also his dignity, is now being defined by theologians according to the belief that human beings were made in God's image, as described in the first chapter of Genesis. However, specific characteristics identifying us as individuals, such as intelligence or self-awareness, or, to be precise, self-respect, make a human being a human being when combined. Conversely, it holds that human dignity is based on a relationship created and made possible by the Creator.[4] Human beings must answer to Him. Stemming from *this* relationship, Man develops four fundamental relationships: to God, to himself, to his fellow men and to all of creation.

The power of the notion that human beings were made in God's image can be seen in the Ten Commandments, in which it states, 'Thou shalt not make unto thee any graven image or likeness' (Exodus 20:4–5, 8). If God cannot be made accessible through an image, which would otherwise mean that he is static and could be worshipped *through* that image, then likewise human beings, who were 'made in

4 In this way, parents' bond to their unborn children is viewed in a larger context, but is not devalued. If God's relationship to His creation is questioned, then other core beliefs of the Christian faith, like the hope of resurrection, are also brought into question.

his image', cannot be made accessible and 'static' (once and for all), but instead they are and remain 'works in progress'.

A human being is limited by the fact that his actions consistently fail to live up to his self-established ideal and his definition of self, which also includes his dignity. In theory, this could lead to a denial of his God-given dignity. However, because this cannot happen, the second axiom of Christian faith is based on the belief that Jesus Christ came to save our sinful, alienated souls. By accepting Him, one expresses a hope for the revocation of this estrangement 'during our limited time on earth and forever in Heaven' and likewise to the *restitutio in integrum*.

Using this approach, Christian ethics can be linked to Kant's Second Formula of the Categorical Imperative, according to which human beings are 'always ends in themselves' and cannot be used as a mere means to another end.

The Christian-based[5] and legally established concept of human dignity (Article 1 of the German Constitution) and the derived concept of protection of life (Article 2, Section 2) are in danger of losing their meaning by being used to address all possible questions. This presumed misuse does not cancel out its good intentions. Rather, we are faced with the challenge of dealing with this basic value of our society in a careful and differentiated way.[6] Relativizing it would be disastrous.[7] I now want to share an excerpt from Bonhoeffer's letters written while in custody, in which he expresses this same insight, though in a different context:

> It is one of the most unbelievable, but at the same time irrefutable experiences … that the basic revocation of God's Commandments in the supposed interest of earthly self-preservation thwarts the very interests of this self-preservation. We can interpret this inadvertent experience in a number of ways. In any case it is certain that from this follows that there are laws governing communal life that are more powerful than anything that aims at rising above them. Therefore, it is not only unjust, but also unwise to ignore these laws … However, it is certain that there is no historically meaningful act that does not exceed the boundaries of these laws at some point. There is, however, a difference between those situations in which the crossing of the established boundary is regarded as the revocation of that law and is, therefore, issued as a particular kind of law, and situations in which the crossing of this boundary remains in our consciousness as an unavoidable fault, and it is justified by the immediate re-establishment and respect of that law and its boundary (Bonhoeffer 2002: 17f.).

2.2 The Goal of Medicine. I suspect that most people here expect that the medical field should 'diagnose, be therapeutic, heal and serve to reduce as well as prevent physical and mental illness' for as many people as possible, thereby making a humane existence possible.[8] In this way, the medical field is structurally conservative. In an

---

5 If one does not share Christian arguments for human dignity, one is then obligated to offer a different logically grounded argument.

6 I agree with Tanner 2002:.27f. on this point.

7 Compare with the arguments Böckenförde presented in his 2003 article, 'Human Dignity was Inviolable. Taking Leave from the Fathers of Our Constitution: New Commentary on Article 1 of the German Constitution Marks a Break with the Past'.

8 PCG 2002: 39. This is because the minimization of pain is the goal of assisted dying. Compare with the Geneva Pledge and the principles according to Paragraph 1 of the

ideal situation, this notion is contrasted with 'designer medicine' (hardly visible in Germany), which seeks to modify human beings in order to produce desired physical traits. This even makes it possible to 'breed' human beings. However, one should not assume that *eo ipso* all who advocate a green light for stem cell research also want a type of 'wish-fulfilling medicine'. However, it is irrefutable that the possibilities offered by biotechnology can be interpreted and used in this way. This can be seen in light of many such concepts and not only in the Anglo-American philosophy, which I illustrate with certain statements by James D. Watson (compare with Watson 2000 and 2001).

2.3 I also suspect that we would all agree that these divisive issues cannot be argued only from a biological–medical point of view, or even less so from an interpersonal, that is, a philosophical–theological, point of view (PCG 2002: 44). These two perspectives depend upon and complement each other, and without the other they would be one-sided, thus wrong.[9]

3. The Catalogue of Questions

The following catalogue of questions takes up older, theological schemata that were developed to warrant an evaluative judgement between life and living pertaining to decisions about life and death in borderline cases.[10] Every controversial issue concerning the matter must be considered with regard to this raster:[11]

3.1 The people as objects which are acted upon and who are affected by controversial

---

professional guidelines for MDs in Germany (100th Congress of German Doctors 1997).

9 Occasionally, one finds also a difference of opinion regarding methods between ethics of principles and consequences. I admit that I cannot extract that much from this debate because all considerations about possible consequences must assess the objectives and side-effects. At least one axiomatically preset value is needed because no system can work without that. Conversely, all principles must be translated into concrete guidelines for behaviour. We must also identify exactly what the principle of potential therapy allows. If concrete and real consequences are not considered and not evaluated, the violations would have to be accepted.

10 I use components from several other arguments, for example by Volz (1998), quoted by Kollek (2001) and Haspel (2002: 144f.). Volz is relevant inasmuch as he critically–constructively examines the criteria for the doctrine of a justified war. These criteria can be extracted from the concrete object (the justified war) and can be applied to other domains. See also Tanner 2002: 26.

11 For the many problems and their contexts, see also the closing report of the Enquête Commission 3/1 of the Thuringia State Parliament, 'Preservation of Human Dignity in Borderline Cases' (DS 3/3854), released on 24 November 2003. The special votes in Parliament reveal the neuralgic points of the debate.

decisions made about research and health policy.

3.2 The people and groups concerned with the decisions in question and about their interests and motives; that is, the subjects. We must be allowed to ask questions about what kinds of interests, besides charitable intentions, are driving research and policy. Or, more explicitly: what role, if at all, are economic interest and debates about the economic conditions allowed to play in the interpretation of the basic values of our constitution?[12]

3.3 Determination of the legitimate authorities, who should, can or have the power to preside over, approve, permit or forbid with regard to decisions made in this field.

3.4 The basic norms, their weaknesses and their systematic relationship and classification.

3.5 The aims of such research and technology. That concerns the openly declared objectives as well as those not declared. To complement this, the aims and motives of those opposed to such technology must also be brought into question.[13]

3.6 The relative nature of the methods. Does more ethically unproblematic research exist, such as work with adult stem cells or the development of other kinds of therapies? As a society, we simply cannot use every possible means to reach certain goals. For example, we have found agreement about the boundaries for organ transplantation, even though the number of available organs remains very limited.

3.7 Consideration of what might be considered a reasonable outlook for success. Society has a right to demand accountability with regard to cost and output in the face of several well-known failures in the area of gene therapy.

3.8 The contexts in which this debate is taking place and with which it interacts. This concerns contexts such as research and historical thinking, the political and economic influences on research, and the set conditions of the legal framework, such as the high public expectations regarding biomedicine and indeed medicine itself, and how they fluctuate.

3.9 The possible damage to our judicial system. If argumentations concerning human dignity such as the interpersonal example or the principle that states that research

---

12 Compare with Hubert Markl's point of view. He sees the debate about whether or not embryos are made in God's image as a luxury that Germany, as a leader in science, cannot afford.

13 The statements of leading theologians of the PCG are often alleged to have unspoken interests. Up to this point, where these interests could be found I have not come across any indication that raises this objection. The fact that academic theologians have a legitimate and fundamental interest in keeping their status as a recognized academic discipline and voice is in view of a widespread scientism neither surprising nor blameworthy. However, it shows what they are interested in.

> freedom has priority over the protection of life in cases of doubt are established as valid legal interpretations, this could have serious, far-reaching consequences.

It is clear that in this short article I cannot deal with all nine points of this complex catalogue of questions. However, I hope that this catalogue or some other will open up an inquiry into ethical opinion-building processes so that the debate will not always be argued with just a few narrow points.

Each of these questions will have to be internally differentiated. Some have even developed into disciplines in their own right, and I shall present one such typical example.

At the same time, I would like to make it clear that I do not presuppose that one single, conclusive argument can be used to give adequate answers to all controversial questions in the biotechnology domain.

The value of these questions, or rather the answers, is varied. Some of them present necessary conditions that have to be fulfilled in order to reach a point of sufficient security and adequacy of the decision desired. Others, particularly the last (3.9), must be considered although they evade clear classification in light of political decisions that are being lobbied for or have just been made.

4. Example: the Question About Those Affected

As much as I endeavoured systematically to bring the relevant questions to light, I alone cannot answer or cope with all of them. That means that what now follows are only representative comments about question 3.1 from a particularly Protestant point of view. They have to be seen as proviso with regard to my reflections and should also indicate how the other points would need to be dealt with.

Very different groups with very diverse legitimate rights are figured into this rubric:

4.1 I start out with the patients, who have an unquestionable right to medical treatment with the best possibility for success in the aforementioned sense of the word. However, it is disputed whether all patients can be lumped together into a single group that is interested solely in advances in medicine and biotechnology as such. In order not to deteriorate into paternalistic argumentation models, I now quote Ina Praetorius, who is an ethicist and has MS:

> There are both healthy and sick hard-line critics of medical high tech. Being sick does not lead inevitably to a single attitude towards all developments that could possible lead to a cure. Just like healthy people, sick people are in a position to think objectively about which 'advances' are desirable for the public welfare and which are not (Praetorius 2001: 56).

This does not mean that one must renounce the right to medical treatment as described above. However, this right must be discussed with those affected in light of the debate about alternatives and treatment variations. Even variations in research methods must be examined. We must also consider the relativeness of the means and of those affected.

4.2 Reflections about the handicapped are in many ways very similar, because a handicap is not only a medical situation, but also a social construct upon which changing valuations about a life as someone handicapped have an effect. I present this here with great caution. The amount of prudence required here alone to act draws attention to the debate about a possible list of PID grounds for abortion. As far as I understand, experts rightly reject discussing openly a specific list of symptom profiles, because affected persons see this as a tendency to eradicate not only a disease, but also the people who suffer from it. However, this impression is not the result of subjective oversensitivity that can be tactfully ignored; rather, it has a strong hold on prevalent social attitudes towards handicapped people. At the same time, no ethics commission could avoid having to come confidentially to an agreement about this list.

4.3 Women who are involved in biotechnological, or rather medical, processes make up the next group of people affected. On the one hand, they are needed as egg donors, and procedures for extracting eggs are expensive, taxing on the body, and risky. On the other hand, they are treated for infertility with procedures in reproduction medicine.[14] The fact that the embryo is dependent on the mother in a symbiotic way makes it necessary to take the mother into account, at least to some extent. As illustrated by PND practices, women are usually examined thoroughly from a technical point of view, yet the subsequent consultation and follow-up (social) care are insufficient because they do not treat each woman as a whole person.[15]

4.4 I shall now move on to a group which is affected directly by such decisions, namely the researchers involved. However, they need to be dealt with in light of the second point (3.2); that is, as the persons who are acting, and their interests and

---

14 What is questionable and debatable here is the ever-growing and strengthening belief in the right to have a child; that is, a healthy child. Apart from the latent illusion that biotechnological means could potentially fulfil such a demand, at this point we must also ask about the distribution of resources in the health system and society's legal responsibility for such treatments. These questions should be differentiated and discussed, on the one hand, in a complex of questions about the relativeness of the means and, on the other hand, in a chapter about the social contexts. The chapter about reasonable outlook for success is also relevant in this case.

15 In light of this, I cannot hold back a self-critical comment about the academic system: it is not at all easy to combine career and family in our academic system, but it is not like this just in Germany. The majority of post-doc positions require voluntary academic celibacy. In cases where not only women but also men have found relatively secure appointments, how old are they? Statistics about childless academicians speak for themselves. I do not know of any sociological studies about the social composition of couples undergoing fertility treatments. However, suspicions point to an academic clientele. Without wanting to argue in a monocausal manner, I fear that a problem supported by the social construction of science is being fought with scientific means.

motives. They are included in this chapter because intervention by those outside the research domain is threatening their freedom to research as guaranteed by Article 5, Section 3 of the German Constitution. With this, a valuable good is also in jeopardy. The freedom of research is not legally constrained.[16] Thus, it can be defined only within the boundaries of the German Constitution. Because the protection of life alone can serve as a sufficient argument for a research ban, it also helps to explain why the debate about protecting the life of in vitro fertilized ova and their pre-nidation development is so fervent and difficult. The Embryo Protection Law regulates such a ban on research.

4.5 We have now come to the last group I would like to mention, namely the objects at the centre of this research, the fertilized egg cells, which are called 'embryos' according to the Embryo Protection Law. In this case, what is disputable has to do with whether or not the embryos have a claim to protection. This is true even in instances where there is no longer a possibility for implantation and continued development. I cannot add anything new to the arguments exchanged here, so instead I shall outline the problems and arguments I think are important.

Exactly when life begins is biologically defined in a number of ways. The beginning of life with the fusion of egg and sperm cell has been attacked as 'biologism' in the Protestant community. I do not find this argument convincing, because every other definition must also use concrete biological criteria to draw the line somewhere. However, because human dignity, or rather the right to protection, is always a question of evaluative attribution and does not stem automatically from empirical data, this point of reference does not really help us. Instead, claims to possible cures stand in opposition to other claims for the protection of the lives of the unborn.

If theological, canonical and civil rights traditions are going to be used to substantiate that human life begins with the joining of egg and sperm cells and become a *new* ecumenical dogma of Church leaders (Tanner 2002: 27), then I need to make an important correction: first of all, the biblical tradition, which from time immemorial recognizes the care God gives to the mother's womb (compare with 1 Jer. and Ps. 139). Moreover, Ottfried Höffe claims that 'the law and morals have always recognized the status and rights of the unborn' (Höffe 2001: 11). Furthermore, according to the civil code, the line of succession has always been determined by the exact moment of possible conception.

The inquiry into whether or not an 'embryonic human' exists at the moment of fertilization keeps the mother's (essential) role in mind and cannot, therefore, be reduced to a mere semantic exercise. Nevertheless, other attempts to define another moment in time or developmental stage at which point a fertilized ovum can be called a 'human embryo' have not been convincing because these supposed objectively predetermined moments discredit each other (compare with Huber 2002b: 38–47). At none of the possible stages of becoming an individual can the fact be ignored that this is a process, which is indeterminate in the beginning stages. However, because

16 In the GDR, the lack of religious freedom went hand in hand with a lack of freedom in the sciences.

PID and its interest in embryonic stem cells start right at this point, namely where and at what point the genetic programme for the forthcoming individual is present, I do not see how we can get away from potentiality and continuity arguments with regard to potential persons.

If the protection of life begins at this decisive moment, then it should have priority over the possibility of finding hypothetical cures. As far as I know, this corresponds also to the standard decision in ethical cases of uncertainty. Normally, the decision is made in favour of life and not potential use.

In this way, I am urging for a tutioristic attitude towards the unborn.

The discussion needs to proceed to the subsequent points, in which merely the questions are often provoking because they analyze the conditions needed for *recta intentio*, for example. However, this must be put aside for a follow-up discussion.

Bibliography

Anselm, R and **Körtner, U.H.J.** (eds) (2003) *Streitfall Biomedizin – Urteilsfindung in christlicher Verantwortung*, Göttingen: Vandenhoeck & Ruprecht

Böckenförde, E.-W. (2003) 'Die Würde des Menschen war unantastbar – Abschied von den Verfassungsvätern – Die Neukommentierung von Artikel I des Grundgesetzes markiert einen Epochenbruch', *Frankfurter Allgemeine Zeitung*, **3**(September), 33–5

Bonhoeffer, D. (2002) *Widerstand und Ergebung – Briefe und Aufzeichnungen aus der Haft. 17. aktualisierte Auflage*, Gütersloh: Gütersloher Verlags-Haus

EKD (eds) (2002) *Im Geist der Liebe mit dem Leben umgehen –Argumentationshilfe für aktuelle medizin- und bioethische Fragen – Ein Beitrag der Kammer für Öffentliche Verantwortung der EKD*, Frankfurt am Main: Gemeinschaftswerk der Evangelischen Publizistik

Haspel, M. (2002) *Friedensethik und Humanitäre Intervention – Der Kosovo-Krieg als Herausforderung evangelischer Friedensethik*, Neukirchen-Vluyn: Neukirchener.

Höffe, O. (2001) 'Rechtspflichten vor Tugendpflichten – Das Prinzip Menschenwürde im Zeitalter der Biomedizin', *Frankfurter Allgemeine Zeitung*, **31** *March*, 11

Huber, W. (ed.) (2002a) *Der gemachte Mensch – Christlicher Glaube und Biotechnik*, Berlin: Wichern-Verlag

Huber, W. (2002b) 'Stufen des Lebensschutzes?', in *Huber (2002a),* 38–47

Knüppel, R. (2001) 'Aktuelle bioethische Fragen in der kirchlichen Diskussion', *Kirchliches Jahrbuch*: Lieferung 1. Dokumente zum kirchlichen Zeitgeschehen, 38–88

Kollek, R. (2001) 'Von der Gentherapie zur Keimbahnmanipulation? Eine Bilanz nach zehn Jahren experimenteller Genübertragung am Menschen', in F. Crüsemann (ed.), *Menschenwürde und biotechnischer Fortschritt im Horizont theologischer und sozialethischer Erwägungen (= Sonderheft Evangelische Théologie, 61), München: Kaiser, 22–48*

Körtner, U., and **Bünker, M.** (2002) *Verantwortung für das Leben – Eine evangelische Denkschrift zu Fragen der Biomedizin – Im Auftrag des Evangelischen*

Oberkirchenrates Augsburgischen und Helvetischen Bekenntnisses, Frankfurt am Main: Gemeinschaftswerk der Evangelischen Publizistik

Praetorius, I. (2001) 'Das "Trumpf-Argument" – und seine Widerlegung', in F. Crüsemann (ed.), *Menschenwürde und biotechnischer Fortschritt im Horizont theologischer und sozialethischer Erwägungen (= Sonderheft Evangelische Théologie, 61), München: Kaiser, 56–60*

Tanner, K. (2002) 'Der menschliche Embryo – ein embryonaler Mensch?' *epd-Dokumentation*, 9, 26–31

Volz, F.-R. (1998) 'Ethik als kritische Theorie des Ethos – eine Skizze zu einigen Aufgaben ethischer Theoriebildung', *Public Health Forum*, 6, 22ff.

Watson, J.D. (2000) *'Die Ethik des Genoms', Frankfurter Allgemeine Zeitung*, **26** (September), 55

Watson, J.D. (2001) *Interview*, in *Süddeutsche Zeitung Magazin*, **1** *June*, 28–33

Chapter Seven

Ethical and Theological Challenges to Human Biotechnology: Observations from the Perspective of Catholic Theology

Joachim Wanke

The current public debate about the prospects and boundaries of modern biotechnological sciences seems to be divided into two standpoints. On the one side, scientists are publicizing the tremendous opportunities proffered by this branch of modern science. On the other side, there is the Church and its ethical objections to pre-natal interventions, particularly in the earliest stages of development. Ultimately, this kind of situation is frustrating, though not because it has to do with power or influence. Rather, it is frustrating because in a democracy technical, scientific and moral questions have to be answered concurrently. The goal is to create a humane culture, which not only makes medical advances available to the general public (and hopefully not just to those who can afford them), but also protects people from instrumentalization and technical manipulation.

I shall present my thoughts about the theme of this conference in four steps.

1. The Increasing Need for Legal and Moral Normative Regulation

Interfering with human life in its earliest stages of development is the result of and a part of modern biomedical technologies. New knowledge in the bioscience domain and the resulting new technological possibilities have created an increasing need for ethical and legal accompaniment because of the extent to which they can interfere with human life. This interference takes away the protection nature is supposed to provide. I am also aware, however, that nature does not only protect, but can also be a threat. To counterbalance this lack of protection, cultural – that is, legal and ethical – compensations are required. This is because as our increasing scientific expertise and the accompanying technical advances present us with more possibilities for manipulating human life at its earliest stages, at the same time these advances yield a growing number of questions regarding which new procedures could be constructive and beneficial and which are simply too risky. Ethical debates and legal measures are the means through which these questions can be answered. It should also be mentioned that 'risky' in this context is used to denote not only procedures that could conceivably be damaging to a person's health, but also those that do not correspond with moral and legal standards for the protection of life, and this is essential for the peaceful formation of an egalitarian culture.

Up to this point, the legal protection of human embryos has focused on linking work with embryos with reproductive medicine (compare with the Embryo Protection Law from 1990/91). The corresponding keyword is in vitro fertilization (IVF). Nevertheless, I shall point out the objections that the Catholic Church has to IVF, which, for example, are also related to the problem of surplus embryos. Today, it turns out that work with embryos, or better yet, interference, clearly satisfies a different need than the one expressed in the past. The donation of embryos, the extraction of stem cell lines, and therapeutic cloning are methods that go way beyond the realm of infertility therapy. If it is possible to help people with serious and incurable diseases with the treatments developed by means of embryonic research, then it could also be possible that democratic society will be pushed to the limit of its balanced value system in dealing with current conflicts with regard to advances in modern medicine. If it turns out that potentially momentous cures cannot be found without damage to human life in its earliest stages, then we are truly being faced with an ethical and legal normative dilemma.

It would probably be too simple to dismiss this challenge with reference to the fact that the protection of life has priority over the duty to provide medical assistance, even though this differentiation has lasting value. From the perspective of Catholic theology, the real problem is the resulting change in the legal structure, which is in turn based on the principle of respect for human dignity. The fact alone that human beings are a species that have a natural inclination to freedom, reason and autonomy was, according to the concept of human rights, developed during the Enlightenment, and our understanding of a modern constitutional state is the basis for an 'equalization' law, which should be valid for all persons. During the Middle Ages, such a law was completely subjugated because of the classification and subordination system that existed at the time.

Modern human biotechnology seems to retreat from this insight. Neither social factors nor the privileges of money and power are supposed to determine the differences, but rather biological traits. Degrees of epigenetic differentiation are being named to relativize the principle of equality. The gradual protection of life is starting to tie protection of life itself to the existing phases of differentiation that occur in the span of a human life. In this way, some claim that an instrumentalized interference with human life is justified.

2. Theological Grounds for Scepticism

Theological scepticism with regard to such views is not so much based on a metaphysical understanding of the processes that take place at the beginning of life, though it would be better than one based on scientific knowledge. Consistent with a theological understanding, the problem goes much deeper than this. Needless to say, the theological expression 'a human being from the very beginning' is a metaphor of sorts. An embryo takes part in life differently than a human being who has already been born. However, the term 'person' must always be used at the various stages of development, albeit in different ways. We already do this with regard to the various stages of life one experiences after birth. For example, a child is a person, but in a different way than a mature adult. The elderly may lose many of their physical and mental competences, but they remain 'persons' until the end of their life.

The problem is that a moral and legal assessment of the status of embryos bound to a differentiation scale can both logically and psychologically lead to a point at which the stages of life are principally unprotected. If biological traits become the basis of moral and legal norms, then eventually other stages must be assessed in a similar way. Ultimately, the fact of the 'consumer' use of nascent human embryos leaves open why this degree of differentiation is allowed to be cited or used and what function might legitimize this kind of instrumentalization. Open-ended legal terms, which would like to change the existing criteria for the protection of embryos in order to reach 'lofty scientific goals', are intentionally imprecisely and generally worded. I now ask the scientists, what gives us the right – ethically and legally – to breach the fundamental principle of the non-instrumentalization of human existence? Does the problem lie in the fact that the embryo is still so small? Or is it something else? Human life is ubiquitously marked by functions that do not exist or are already deteriorating. And one can be sure that the demand will be that one treat other human 'beings' with the same equality. This is also thought to be true if they, for whatever reason, cannot or partially cannot develop the potential for reason-based self-determination. In other situations, a human countenance is barely recognizable because of disease and deterioration. And the abilities and rational qualities of humankind are also thought to be permanently under threat.

With that in mind, my main concern will be addressed in the third section.

3. Respect for Human Existence for Its Own Sake

The notion of equality, which follows from the discovery of the principle of human dignity in the Christian tradition and the Enlightenment, is anchored more deeply and is of a different moral quality than what mere biological qualification of human life can offer. In order to understand human dignity as an unquestionable value, as Immanuel Kant does, one cannot simultaneously grant it more to some 'beings' and less to others. It is difficult to anchor the guarantee of human dignity in the legal balancing of controversially linked basic rights and likewise to bring the legal issues (for example, medical progress) to the forefront. We cannot conclude from this dilemma that the guarantee of human dignity is a completely empty norm that has a concrete profile only in light of finding a balance within our basic rights. In the context of German constitutional interpretation, the concrete contents of human dignity's normativity are construed as a human being's 'existence for its own sake' (German Constitutional Court 88, 203: 252).

> This includes status and recognition as a subject of its own, the freedom of personal development, the exclusion of instrumentalization as a kind of disposable object (Böckenförde 2003: 811f.).[1]

Therefore, in light of developments in modern human biotechnology and medicine, theology is urging us not to be too hasty in making the structure of rights based on the principle of human dignity flexible. It wants to steer the research in the direction of developing new procedures out of consideration for thc normative dimensions of modern culture, which would not be so taxing on the development of nascent embryos. It would also be conceivable to work more with the extraction of adult stem cells or procedures for extracting embryonic stem cells that do not destroy the embryos, which future research still has to substantiate. If these less dramatic developments are not possible or not desired, then our culture based on human rights will be in considerable distress. Therefore, we need to keep in mind the risks and shortcomings of such practices, which need to be overcome not only with scientific–technical solutions, but also with better moral solutions.

4. Closing Remarks About Some Ideological Implications

The public debate about the capabilities of new discoveries in human biotechnology is not about conflicts of fact. In contrast to earlier times during which scientific knowledge collided with faith-based interpretations of the world – keyword, Galileo – the problem today has to do with questions of ethical interpretation. These problems can be solved only when we try to make sense of the interpretations.

Technical knowledge that is available to experts always falls short of the complexity of human life, and it can put a strain on our lives if it begins to dominate the actions of society. In the eyes of the Catholic Church, pre-natal diagnosis, which is carried out in correlation with our knowledge of human genetics, is an example of the one-sided exaggeration of human actions. Furthermore, many parents feel overwhelmed by this experience. Even though the line between diagnostic possibilities and therapeutic capabilities may not be so clear in the future (which we all hope), our society is using the knowledge we have already gained to destroy human life, not to heal it. In this way, modern research can have an excluding effect.

In view of possible modifications to the human genome, which will likely be practicable in the future, the following statement is valid: what is changed by manipulation in the earliest stages of human life has an effect on the entire person. For this reason, pre-natal stages of development (even very early on) cannot be separated from the life of the person. Criticism of a naturalistic point of view, which does not take into account the progressive character of embryonic development, does not address the concerns of the Catholic Church. Additionally, those who propose other qualitative, in-between steps still have to take this progressive character into account. In my opinion, it is fair to maintain that human life begins with the fusion of egg and sperm cell, despite unanswered questions. This docs justice to the concepts

1 E.-W. Böckenförde (2003) 'Menschenwürde als normatives Prinzip – Die Grundrechte in der bioethischen Débatte', *Juristische Zeitung*, 58, 809–15.

of potentiality and continuity. Therefore, from a biological perspective, it would be correct to say that a human being in the early stages of development is just a mass of cells, but it is not inaccurate when one takes into account the existence of genetic information and the significance of the cell mass for epigenetic development. The protection granted to a nascent human embryo cannot be decreased in order to fulfil the objectives of stem cell research. We cannot lose our intuition that the embryo phase is part of human life in its completeness and part of the inviolability of human dignity.

Theological thought refuses to accept a view of human beings that relegates them to mere raw material during certain phases of their development. Respect for the miracle of life, which modern science will never be able to fully grasp or get to the bottom of, remains a necessary, cultural and society-shaping value. Scientific thought and intervention simply cannot entirely overlook this. It overtaxes itself and in the end leaves only disappointment behind. It might also be good to occasionally relativize our definition of 'advancement'. Johann Nestroy once said, 'Progress looks much bigger than it really is.'

The safe-guarding and peace-making quality of moral boundaries which maintains that no individual can be sacrificed for the interests of others must be understood to reside at the symbolic–normative core even in the earliest stages of human development. The acknowledgement of such a boundary makes both the humane construction of an ideological pluralistic society and democratic consensus possible. Therefore, this concern is in the same way an issue at the end of life. Purely technical answers to questions about uncertainties with regard to dying with dignity fail to see the challenge of truly humane assisted dying. Models for active euthanasia seem to comply with our society's need for self-determination. In reality, however, they replace the general psycho-social commitment to people in the last phase of their life with a pain-free death. In contrast to this, a humane death calls for holistic care and solidarity, not desolidarization, which also burdens the dying person with having to make the decision to die.

A faith-based interpretation of the world has a feel for the sanctity of human life. To recall and remember the last mystery of human life is not an irrational demand; rather, it is consistent with the reality of our existence. The Christian faith pits this view of human life against the unrealistic demand for complete control of nature through technology and science. The need to accept suffering, to learn how to live with it, and to give it meaning is, along with the strategies that aim to conquer life's shortfalls through science and technology, an ever-present and important dimension of our culture. Those who misleadingly push only one biased or polarized aspect of this debate into the foreground put a big strain on us all. Some scientific domains are currently in danger of promising therapies even though they have not yet developed the necessary methods. The ethical and theological challenge facing human biotechnology exists in the reminder to be realistic, honest and modest.

PART IV
Philosophical and Theological Ethics

Chapter Eight

Human Dignity as a Regulatory Principle of Bioethics: A Theological Perspective

Reiner Anselm

The current bioethical debate can be characterized by two diverging tendencies. First, reductionist intervention with regard to the normative concepts used in the assessment of this problem (see also Huber 1994 and 2002) is faced with the unremitting differentiation of the description of ethical problems. Furthermore, this is accompanied by the further development of descriptive–hermeneutic methods in the field of ethics (to find the source of this concept in Protestant theological ethics, compare with the model in Fischer 2002). This gap between description and assessment, which, in theory, should be closed by an application-orientated ethics (see also Nida-Rümelin 1996), instead seems to be growing even wider. However, an awareness of the correlation between scientific knowledge and ethical assessment has increased in the last few years, particularly in the field of bioethics. *Feminis*t critique on traditional ethical theoretical models has made it even more clear that ethics is very much contingent on its context. Nonetheless, efforts to find a context-sensitive appraisal in the field of ethics are at odds with attempts to establish a standardized normative concept. The almost extreme overuse of the term 'human dignity' in the current bioethical debate is the result of this attempt. At the same time, this illustrates the problem German-speaking ethicists and philosophers have had in forming new theories that seek to find an adequate and definitive basis for ethical judgements. This is to be understood as an attempt to integrate discrete societal values and application domains.

Descriptive and normative elements of the bioethical debate are unexpectedly in opposition to one another. Furthermore, it is the dynamics of change in the scientific–technical domain itself that allows the emphasis on one side or the other to appear justified. On the one hand, advances in science are accompanied with an increase in possible procedures and methods, and with that comes also the need to keep an eye on these situations and their inherent conflicts. Ethical reflection is made up, for the most part, of an adequate description of these application-orientated contexts, because decision-makers must first know what they are talking about before they can act. In this case, ethics represents a differentiation of perception. It also signifies a methodically controlled process, in which possibilities and risks are weighed against each other. This process is in itself also a part of the dynamics of progress. On the other hand, in the search for action-guiding points of orientation, we can also observe an opposing process within the scope of ethical reflection. The impulse to strive towards a reduction of complexity is fundamentally related to the criteria for human dignity, which have found wide acceptance in recent bioethical debates. The confusing diversity of ethical practice should be contrasted with the orientating clarity of a 'superordinating term'. This corresponds to the fact that the call for 'ethics' is often a nuanced criticism of modernity. In this instance, ethics denotes a cipher for a concept of social homogeneity that has been lost in the process of modernization, or at the very least one can say that its existence is threatened and without it social co-existence no longer seems possible. Nevertheless, despite this subliminal or sometimes explicit critique on modernity, these concepts remain firmly bound to the ideals of the Enlightenment and the modern age.

Presently, a new interest in the relationship between religion and ethics makes this clear, but this interest needs to be evaluated. So far has it been acknowledged that the desired integration can only result from a perceived transcendental ideal. Thereby, the function-orientated intervention that is characteristic of the modern age becomes evident. In this debate, religion and its symbols no longer maintain their legitimacy through a revelation-based concept of God, but instead through their *usefulness* for society. Religion is ascribed a stabilizing function for maintenance of an ideal of humanity whose recognition as such is purportedly safeguarded only in instances in which it remains tightly bound to absolute values. A good place to observe this structure is in reflections about the principle of human dignity. The correlation of the concept of human dignity with long-standing reflections about the belief that human beings were created in God's image, which stems from the Creation stories in the Judaeo-Christian tradition, is, on the one hand, based on an interest to provide the principle of human dignity with a stable, religiously metaphysical foundation. On the other hand, this is also characteristic of the modern age's functional access to the continued existence of religion as a whole. Since Émile Durkheim and possibly before, religion has been considered to be an 'essentially collective affair' (Durkheim 1981: 68), which is characterized primarily by a 'system of convictions and practices' and can be the catalyst for the emergence of a 'moral community' (Durkheim 1981: 68). All of the great sociologists after Durkheim, from Max Weber to Talcott Parsons, have argued in a similar way. Currently, the leading philosophers of post-traditional and post-metaphysical theories have an increasingly louder voice. Despite a well-cultivated secularization theory, they ascribe religion to an essential societal role. According to Jürgen Habermas,[1] this is because religion guarantees the emergence of those values that are requisite for collective co-existence. From this perspective, the principle of human dignity serves as the equivalent to a transcendental, metaphysically based supreme argument within the scope of ethics.

---

1 Jürgen Habermas emphasized his high regard for religion as a functioning social structure again in a speech during the awards ceremony for the German Book Trade's Prize for Peace. In this speech, he also amended the ideal of a 'post-traditional ethos': 'In view of the religious roots of its moral foundations, the liberal state should expect the possibility that the "culture of collective human reason" (Hegel) will not catch up with the level of the description of its genesis, particularly in view of the new challenges. Today, the language of the market seeps into every pore and presses all relationships between people into a schema of self-centred orientation. However, the social band, which is linked to mutual recognition, is not wrapped up in the terms of the contract, rational choice, and the maximization of use' (Habermas 2001: 23); see Habermas 1992: 129 for an explanation of 'post-traditional ethos'.

However, with such an affinity between ethics and religion as a backdrop, it seems doubtful that the concept of human dignity can actually reach the goals ascribed to it, such as the reduction of complexity as well as the integration of conflicting circumstances and values. Reflections about the concept 'religion' and about God can help us see that such concepts aimed at integration are always bound to concrete historical developments. *Ideas* about God develop an orientating power not as something abstract, but rather only when they are related to a story, for example the story of the chosen people of Israel or the life, death and resurrection of Jesus Christ. Today, of course, the stories themselves no longer appear to be manifestations of *history in general*, but instead are solitary narratives. As both solitary and potentially polemogenic stockpiles, they themselves require the integration of a concept of unity or of God derived by reason – at least, according to the insights of early modern religious disputes. However, in the struggle to maintain its integrating power, this concept of unity or of God loses it orientating power to the same extent in that it is detached from the concrete contexts to which it owes its existence. From theory's ivory tower, the differences down below may seem meaningless; however, orientation problems do not originate in lofty theories, but instead in lowly spheres of everyday life. As early as 1799, Friedrich Schleiermacher made mention of this in his essay 'Discussing Religion': 'If a religion is not supposed to be a specific one, then it is not a religion at all, but rather it is a collection of loosely constructed, unrelated things' (Schleiermacher 1799/1991: 186). The responsibilities of theology, which are both unique and interminable, have always comprised both the mediation between transcendence and immanence, and the efforts to allow the Hereafter to profit from conditions in this life, though without putting earthly existence in the place of our existence in the Hereafter and without passing off history as metaphysics.

The principle of human dignity is under similar pressure. It is also considered to be a construct that should serve as an instrument of integration in the face of a myriad of conflicting values and norms. Nevertheless, much like the concepts of religion and God, it can only be realized when it is abstracted from a concrete historical-based view of human dignity. This means, however, that 'human dignity' is just an empty phrase. With this in mind, we are now faced with a paradoxical situation: as an integrating power, human dignity can only develop as an empty formula, that is, as an 'un-interpreted theory', which Theodor Heuss discussed during the German Constitution Council of 1949.[2] The concept of human dignity can lay claim to its orientating quality only if it can renew the support of a particular tradition of interpretation – and then, of course, only at the cost of a more specific 'follow-up capacity'. At present, these two aspects are often obscured or disregarded. For this reason, it is advisable to reposition reflections about human dignity in the ethical debate. When we take a closer look, it becomes clear that the human dignity argument in no way represents the normative counterpoint to a descriptive, method-based ethics. Instead, both concepts behave more as complements.

In my opinion, more attention needs to be dedicated to a more exact description of the traditions that drive the orientating ability of the principle of human dignity.

---

2 Theodor Heuss discusses his recommendation for the formulation of Article 1, Section 1 of the German Constitution, as quoted in Doemming, Füßlein & Matz 1951: 49.

Only when we answer for the implications of having individual interpretations of the term 'human dignity' can we counteract the danger of absolutizing our own opinions. From this perspective, we must resist the temptation of turning 'human dignity' into a Trojan horse by which other maxims and ideals can be smuggled into the decision-making process (compare with Ehmke & Schneider 1963: 83; also with Maihofer 1968: 88; Denninger 1973: 23). What is more, only on the basis of the historization of the concept of human dignity can we understand why reference to 'human dignity' in no way *ends* ethical debates, but instead *opens* them.

I would now like to present a general picture of two different traditions. In Graeco-Roman classical antiquity, as well as in the traditions of the Renaissance, Humanism and the Enlightenment, the historical development of the concept of human dignity is very tightly bound to the realization that humankind's dignity lies in the traits that distinguish it from other life forms. In particular, it resides in man's indeterminable nature and in his ability to reason. Reflections about human dignity in both the Bonn Constitution and Charter of the UN have their roots in this tradition. Accordingly, it states in Article 1 of the Universal Declaration on Human Rights, 'All human beings are born free and equal in dignity and rights. They are endowed with reason and conscience and should act towards one another in a spirit of brotherhood.' It is obvious that the right to life, human dignity and the ability to reason are correlated here. It should not be hard to see that this close association could prove to be dysfunctional in light of the challenges brought about by advances in medicine and in the biosciences. In the current public debate in the field of medical ethics, the focus is on protecting the lives of those who for one reason or another do not have the abilities of reason, self-awareness, self-reflection, self-determination or communication. This is true for the unborn as well as the severely handicapped, comatose, brain-dead and those suffering from dementia. In all of these cases, reference to human dignity should (as a rule) guarantee physical existence and freedom from bodily harm, independent of a human being's state of development at any given moment.

In order to reach this point, another interpretation model for the human dignity argument is needed. It is characterized by the fact that it does not make dignity dependent on any intrinsic characteristics, but instead it begins with the statement that human dignity is *ascribed* to every human being. For this reason, it is in no way accidental that this argumentation plays an especially important role in the opinions of Church and theologians. Furthermore, this is established irrespective of theological and denominational differences about a suitable correlation between theological concepts and the concept of human dignity. In the Protestant Church, for example, the awareness that human beings have dignity not from within, as an inborn quality or ability, but rather that it comes from God alone has always been present. The opinion that the abilities of reason and self-governance are anthropologically founded has been very critically questioned in both the Protestant and Roman Catholic traditions.

From this standpoint, if we see how much the normative and explicative content of the principle of human dignity depends on a preceding traditional framework, then we can incisively state that human dignity is not a normative concept in its own right, but rather it represents a cipher for the presence of ethics in debates which not only address advances in biomedicine, but also general questions about the structure of society. In ethical conflict situations, the orientating ability that it ascribes to ethics derives from the fact that the scope of ethical reflection, which is expanded by the principle of human dignity, is filled with elements of prior ethos. Accordingly, the German Constitutional Court also declared:

> Human dignity is something that is not disposable. However, recognizing what the command to respect human dignity requires cannot be separated from history. A judgement regarding what corresponds to human dignity can only be based on the current state of knowledge and cannot lay claim to interminable validity (German Constitutional Court 45, 187: 229).[3]

Human dignity's regulating nature is not based fundamentally in its meaning, but more in the fact that it serves as a *placeholder* for various ethical traditions. For this reason, it can be coupled with a multitude of theoretical- and interpretation-orientated traditions, but the concept itself is in need of interpretation.

Demand for the interpretation of the concept of human dignity has become the latest subject of a passionate legal debate. Matthias Herdegen's new commentary on Article 1, Section 1 of the German Constitution in the standard commentary of the Constitution begun by Theodor Maunz and Günter Dürig is the reason for this (Herdegen 2001 and 2003). According to Dürig, the principle of human dignity serves as the 'basis for an entire value system that at the same time turns out to be a logical system of claims, in which a core value is to the subordinating values as a legal *propositio maior* is to a legal *propositio minor*' (Dürig 1956: 119). Together they project a value system that is endowed to the state, but that deprives the state of its power to regulate. Both are translated into positive law without ever having to be substantiated.

Herdegen continues the interpretation tradition initiated by Dürig and subjects it to a critical revision. According to Herdegen, it cannot originate from an over-positive, pre-government definition of human dignity on the level of *constitutional* interpretation, nor can it be constituted through a hierarchical and unchanging value system. On the contrary, such a value system always needs to be defined anew through the interpretation and evaluation processes of competing basic rights.

Ernst-Wolfgang Böckenförde was vehemently opposed to an interpretation that tried to obliterate the material meaning of the guarantee of human dignity through a plurality of interpretations, and he was ready to abandon the metaphysical foundation of the law as the parenthesis between law and justice. In his treatise 'Human Dignity was Inviolable', which appeared in the newspaper the *Frankfurter Allgemeinen*, he once again tried to pit the 'principle of personality', which is part of Catholic social teachings, against the openness of interpretation of the principle of human

---

3 Compare also with Arthur Kaufmann 2001: 'Human dignity is an abstract concept, without a tangible, definable content. For this reason, one can pretty much apply it to everything. And many do this enthusiastically .... Such an abstract and utterly normative concept like human dignity cannot be logically subsumed. In reality, what one does is include the personal understanding of human dignity. There are many such examples, that what one puts into the human dignity ideas is what one later gets out of it.'

dignity. Böckenförde went on to say that without the foundation of a value system that is incorporated into the constitution, but is also higher than any government action, the legal and social order would be robbed of its keystone. This is because an interpretation of the Constitution carried out in this way can only establish a relative absoluteness. Instead of giving it normative authority for the present, Herdegen shifts the historically based intellectual and cultural roots of the human dignity argument to legal history as 'an intellectual backdrop' of interests without practical relevance. For Böckenfoerde, Article 1 of the Constitution is 'no longer the very foundation and meta-positive embodiment of the constitutional system, no longer the constant in the fluid discourse about constitutional legality, but rather it is entrusted to the community of constitutional interpreters for whom no binding canon for interpretation exists' (Böckenförde 2003: 35).

Despite what the cultural critical–polemical undertone of Böckenförde's writings would like to suggest, the recognition of a need for interpretation in no way indicates that the orientating power of the theorem of human dignity should surrender to its unpredictability and the arbitrariness of the zeitgeist. The fact is that every interpretation, even Böckenförde's alleged meta-positive position, is based on the foundation of what has already been, and upon this foundation it finds its own footings. With his gift of terseness, Odo Marquard sums this up in the following way:

> Only in the fact that given historical facts are always there, as a guideline, do our own efforts have a chance; no one can start from the very beginning, everyone must go on from that which is already there: the future needs the past' (Marquard 1977: 16).

Continuing in Marquard's train of thought, the past as a guideline does not simply replace these 'efforts'. Likewise, linkage is not limited to redundancy, but rather it opens up the future. The reason for Böckenförde's critique might have been one of Herdegen's statements, in which he questions precisely this limiting posterior method of interpretation based on the tradition of a bygone ethos with regard to the debate about embryo protection. Herdegen maintains that with regard to the protection of embryos at the earliest stages of development the point is that 'a dimension of the right to the protection of dignity, which has been the centre of intellectual discourse for the last two and a half thousand years and deals with matters such as the belief that man is made in God's image, the point at which human beings have a soul, moral autonomy and the belief that an individual is an end in itself, offers an equally unreliable approach as the weakly contoured conception of humankind in the German Constitution' (Herdegen 2003: 32). As such, this is undoubtedly correct. For the current debates, no direct, normative conclusion can be derived from the interpretation models of the past or from the belief that human beings are made in God's image. And yet, every opinion that is justifiably formed here in the present has its roots in the theories formed in the past, even when it is anchored to the public discourse about the interpretation of the principle of human dignity. This latter point is clearly favoured by Herdegen. Just as one cannot derive unbroken norms from history, one cannot produce norms in the present without reaching back into the past.

The reason for this is that we always strive for stability and continuity, with regard to our personal biography as well as to our social relationships.

A glimpse into the constitutive historicity of the human dignity debate takes a back seat concerning not only the alternative between a descriptive, application-orientated ethics and a normative, paradigmatic ethics that is orientated on the concept of dignity, but also the correlated question about a metaphysical or positivist foundation for the Article about human dignity. Just as argumentation that would like to base itself on the metaphysical underpinning of the law cannot help admitting that every such statement can present itself only as an historically determined form of expression stemming from a metaphysical argument, a legal-positivistic view must also acknowledge that its own theory-formation process is always influenced by the proviso of topicality. However, the exact contours of this time-based relation are out of reach of the positivistic validation theory. To make the disagreements between Herdegen and Böckenförde clear once again: both argue in ways characteristic for their time, and for this reason there is a counter position against a wide-ranging rhetoric that is generally binding as well as a counter position against a purely arbitrary human dignity argument.

This framework makes it possible to connect discourse about human dignity with belief systems in a new way, which has become characteristic of modern Protestant theology. This is because the task of theology is to make statements about the transcendental and the 'super-historical' under the conditions of historicity and then to interpret them within concrete situations. However, this must be done without losing the transcendental basis of its theory-forming process and its sermonizing function. In 1922, Karl Barth expressed the tension in this formula in the following way:

> As theologians, we are supposed to talk about God. However, we are human beings and as such cannot talk about God. We should know both what we should do and what we cannot do, and through that we can honour God. This is our biggest difficulty. In comparison, everything else is child's play' (Barth 1922: 199).

The task of theology is to mediate between transcendence and immanence, by which transcendence should always appear as a part of immanence, though without losing its lustre or being swallowed up by it. Perhaps it is already discernible in my exposition, that in a particular way this is the task of Christian theology. Jesus Christ, who is true God and true man, represents the mediation between transcendence and immanence. Therefore, the Christian faith traces this tension back to the founder himself. Furthermore, according to Christianity, every proclamation made in the spirit of the Christian faith, in its humanity and temporality, must express God's greatness. I shall try to make this clear with the example of Communion. According to Protestant belief, it is an expression of God's greatness that He associates Himself with the (human) celebration of Communion, but this does not mean that God is identical with the bread and wine; that is, the bread and wine do not become Him. Again, I refer to Karl Barth:

> Our difficulty is our promise .... However, it could be that I do not just say that our difficulty is our promise. It could be that this is a living truth that is greater than yes or no,

> the reality of God, which is not at my disposal through a dialectical reversal that could be accessed with one's own power or love. It could also be that the Word, the Word of God that we will never speak, has taken on our weakness and falseness, so that our word, in its weakness and falseness, would become able to become, at the very least, a container and a sort of vessel for the word of God (Barth 1922: 217f.).

I would now like to take up the aforementioned affinity between Christianity and the principle of human dignity in such a way that I may convert the tension-filled relationship between transcendence and immanence, as discussed in theology, into a postulate of the *relative absoluteness* of the concept of human dignity, which was first introduced by Jack Donnelly (compare with Donnelly 1984: 219). Relative absoluteness should symbolize seeing the human dignity argument's claim to unconditional-ness in the demand for ethical reflection, which acknowledges its own perspectivity as self-limiting and at the same time seeks to dialogically expand, so that it is prepared to fix its orientating power to specific structural conditions.

However, this kind of contextualization does not mean that thoughts about human dignity should surrender to arbitrariness simply for the fact that a bygone ethos is at an individual's disposal as an historically founded authority. Instead, the human dignity argument likens itself to a normative core that exists merely in an appeal not only to view human existence and human actions in a sectoral–monoperspectival way, but to keep them in the foreground so that human beings do not develop in such situations in which simply no sectoral–reductionist equivalent is permitted. Reference to free will as the foundation for *dignitas hominis* in Renaissance philosophy is also related to fundamental principles, such as reference to the ability to reason or the idea that man is one of God's creations. Within this fundamental structure, which has its roots in Rawls's thoughts on 'the balance of reflection' regarding concrete questions of orientation, also lies the reference to the transcendentality of the idea of human dignity.

If this analysis is correct, then it gives rise to other perspectives for the application of the human dignity argument in bioethical debates:

(1) By nature, human dignity is a concept that is always open to interpretation. Its framework points to the fact that possible actions must not be understood as monoperspectival and sectoral. Furthermore, bestowing it with a singular, binding meaning is not permissible. To establish an interpretation of the concept of human dignity means simultaneously destroying the very core of the human dignity argument.

(2) The frequently cited formula that states that human dignity represents the generally accepted frame of reference for ethical discourse turns out to be a (slight) tautology when considered within this context. In the bioethical domain, reference to human dignity, in the first place, means only that ethical questions with regard to biomedical advances are raised at all; for example, in the context of our present-day reality, what is a 'good life'? This is very clear in cases where the term human dignity is used attributively, for example in the search for humane forms of treatment. Furthermore, when we talk about looking for humane therapies, we actually mean options for action, which, because of criteria that go beyond mere scientific–medical findings and validate single facts, take into account the complexity of the decision-making process. Within these processes, technical knowledge is just as important as experience, and the specific experiences of a generation are as significant as ways of thinking. At the same

time, this indicates that reference to human dignity as a criterion forms the beginning, not the end, of ethical discourse. This also explains why the principle of human dignity is not apposite for providing concrete guidelines for action.

(3) Human dignity's regulative function could be said to serve as a vanishing-point for various ethical concepts and to avoid the establishment of a specific interpretation and assessment model. It is true also that through critical analysis, the various ideological implications that are present with reference to reflections about human dignity need to be uncovered and re-introduced within the ethical discourse. From this perspective, ethics is embedded within an extensive historico-cultural research programme.

(4) Within the framework of such an analysis, it might be possible to gain a more precise awareness of areas of overlap between the various ethical concepts within a defined cultural context. In this way, the regulative function of human dignity could be linked with 'basic ethical consensus' or common sense.

(5) More far-reaching definitions cannot be derived consistently from mere reference to reflections about human dignity, in particular with regard to the correlation between human dignity and the modern, enlightened demand for the protection of every individual's freedom. For example, decisions made regarding germ line therapy show that reflections on human dignity cannot easily be restricted to the protection of an individual person. On the contrary, corresponding derivations are due to the respective ideological traditions that form the basis of the argumentation.

(6) From this standpoint, the job of Protestant ethics should be to clarify its respective connection to tradition and its ability to serve the interpretation and concretization of the cipher 'human dignity'. Along these lines, Protestant ethics must also state how specific and core concepts of a Protestant view of reality affect a corresponding interpretation of the concept of human dignity.

Criteria for human dignity capable of reaching consensus can only be found if we can also agree on the understanding of reality that lies at the core. Efforts to reveal such implicit axioms are, in my opinion, an essential prerequisite when the objectives are bound to references to human dignity and to reaching agreement about the attitudes, ideologies and generational experiences that shape them. Protestant theological ethics should concentrate on revealing and analyzing these traditional contexts and giving up the stern tone of a legal sermon. Where could this kind of ethics, which in fact owes itself to the insights of the Reformation, be more impressively laid out than here in the Wartburg Castle?

Bibliography

Barth, K. (1922) 'Das Wort Gottes als Aufgabe der Theologie', in J. Moltmann (ed.) (1977), *Die Anfänge der Dialektischen Theologie*, vol. 1, fourth edn, Kaiser, München, 179–218

Böckenförde, E.-W. (2003) 'Die Würde des Menschen war unantastbar', *Frankfurter Allgemeine Zeitung*, **3**, 33 and 35

Denninger, E. (1973) *Staatsrecht – Einführung in die Grundprobleme des Verfassungsrechts der Bundesrepublik Deutschland*, Reinbek bei Hamburg: Rowohlt

Doemming, K.-B., **Füßlein, R.W.**, and **Matz, W.** (1951) 'Entstehungsgeschichte der Artikel des Grundgesetzes', *JöR NF*, **1**, 41ff.

Donnelly, J. (1984) 'Cultural relativism and universal human rights', *Human Rights Quarterly*, **6**, 400–19 [DOI: 10.2307/762182]

Dürig, G. (1956) 'Der Grundrechtssatz von der Menschenwürde', *AöR*, 81, 117–57

Durkheim, É. (1981) *Die elementaren Formen des religiösen Lebens*, Frankfurt am Main: Suhrkamp

Ehmke, H., and **Schneider, P.** (1963) *Prinzipien der Verfassungsinterpretation*, Berlin: Walter de Gruyter Books

Fischer, J. (2002) *Theologische Ethik – Grundfragen und Orientierung*, Stuttgart et al.: Kohlhammer

Habermas, J. (1992) *Faktizität und Geltung – Beiträge zur Diskurstheorie des Rechts und des demokratischen Rechtsstaates*, Frankfurt am Main: Suhrkamp.

Habermas, J. (2001) *Glauben und Wissen – Friedenspreis des deutschen Buchhandels*, Frankfurt am Main: Suhrkamp

Herdegen, M. (2001) 'Die Menschenwürde im Fluß des bioethischen Diskurses', *JZ*, **56**, 773–9

Herdegen, M. (2003) 'Kommentar zu Art. 1 Abs. 1 GG', in T. Maunz and G. Dürig (eds), *Grundgesetz – Kommentar*, vol. 1, Art. 1–11, München: Beck, 1–58

Huber, W. (1994) 'Grenzen des medizinischen Fortschritts aus ethischer Sicht', *Zee*, **38**, 41–53

Huber, W. (2002) *Der gemachte Mensch – Christlicher Glaube und Biotechnik*, Berlin: Wichern-Verlag

Kaufmann, A. (2001) 'Was der Mensch dem Menschen schuldet', *Süddeutsche Zeitung*, **31** May

Maihofer, W. (1968) *Rechtsstaat und menschliche Würde*, Frankfurt am Main: Klostermann

Marquard, O. (1977) 'Ende des Schicksals? Einige Bemerkungen über die Unvermeidlichkeit des Unverfügbaren', in O. Marquard, J. v.Ess and R. Koselleck (eds), *Schicksal? Grenzen der Machbarkeit – Ein Symposium, München: DTV, 7–25*

Nida-Rümelin, J. (1996) *Angewandte Ethik – Die Bereichsethiken und ihre theoretische Fundierung – Ein Handbuch*, Stuttgart: Kröner

Schleiermacher, F.D.E. (1799/1991) *Über die Religion – Reden an die Gebildeten unter ihren Verächtern*, ed. V.R. Otto, seventh edn, Göttingen: Vandenhoeck & Ruprecht

Chapter Nine

Tolerance and Respect in Bioethical Conflicts

Nikolaus Knoepffler

1. Background

Because of new possibilities in human biotechnology, different convictions often collide often in conflict situations. This is nothing out of the ordinary for a pluralistic society. Therefore, how these convictions are presented and how representatives of other opinions are treated is very significant. I would like to elucidate this with the example of 'pre-implantation diagnosis'. After a brief description of the medical facts and various assessment options, I shall explain why consensus is not possible in this conflict, which means that we are dealing with a test case for tolerance. The description of a well-known viewpoint, which does not respect the other side, will serve as a counter-example to show what form a debate marked by respect and tolerance should take and, consequently, what might make socially workable compromises possible.

2. A Test Case: 'Pre-Implantation Genetic Diagnosis'

2.1. Medical Facts

Pre-implantation genetic diagnosis (PGD) is a new and revolutionary practice in the area of genetic diagnosis (see also Knoepffler 2004: 110–14). It is an invasive, genetic engineering procedure usually performed on an in vitro embryo at the point when it is made up of six to ten cells. Approximately 48–70 hours after a zygote has formed, two cells from the blastomere are removed from the embryo and examined. Depending on the situation, normally one uses either the Polymerase Chain Reaction (PCR), which can diagnose recessive hereditary diseases, or the Fluorescence in situ Hybridization (FiSH), which can identify Trisomy 21, for example. There is the possibility that the individual who has already been born and who developed from an implanted embryo *after* a PGD is at risk also for the imprinting phenomenon (Claussen 2001: 398). This can lead to an increased number of neo-natal complications, and in some cases to reduced growth. In addition to these risks, there are the normal risks and stresses connected with in vitro fertilization (IVF). Over and above that, a misdiagnosis is also possible, even with pre-implantation diagnosis, although the risk is slight (*c*. 3–5 per cent).

What is the primary aim of this diagnosis according to the view of the German Association of MDs (Bundesärztekammer 2000)? It is intended to detect specific genetic mutations that can cause serious diseases before implantation. With regard to spontaneous miscarriages, we assume that a majority of the embryos and foetuses were not going to be capable of surviving because of mutations in the genotype. However, newborns also have a 3–5 per cent risk of having a deformity or disease. Chromosome disorders and monogenic diseases – that is, diseases caused only by one gene sequence – make up about 1.5 per cent of this group. Additionally, the risk of such deformities or diseases rises concurrently with the age of the mother. This increase is not linear; starting at age 36, it escalates very quickly. For example, a 35-year-old woman is four times more likely to have a child with the chromosome Trisomy 21 (Down's syndrome), whereas a 45-year-old woman is 50 times more likely (see also National Ethics Council 2003: 40). This particular chromosome disorder leads to mental handicap and is often the cause of heart defects and other physical problems.

If one or both parents have a high risk for genetic diseases, then the risk that the children will have a chromosome disorder or monogenic disease is calculated differently. For autosomal recessive diseases – that is, genetic changes that are not in the sex chromosomes – there is a 25 per cent risk when both parents are carriers of the disease. One example of this is cystic fibrosis. However, when the recessive change is found in the sex chromosomes, then the situation is a bit different. For example, with haemophilia, which is caused by a change in the X-chromosome, there is a 50–50 risk that boys will have it when the mother is the carrier, even if the father is healthy. If the father has the disease but the mother is not a carrier, then the offspring will not have the disease. None of the male offspring will be carriers, but 50 per cent of the female offspring will be born as carriers.

In the case of autosomal dominant genetic changes, the affected parent – that is, the parent who passes the change on – always has the disease, or rather the disposition, because the defective gene dominates his or her healthy allele. For this reason, offspring with an affected parent have a 50 per cent chance of having the same disease. A classic example of this is Huntington's disease, which typically appears in predisposed patients between the ages of 35–50 and leads to both physical and mental deterioration. This is, without exception, a terminal disease. Through PGD, one has the chance to find out whether the embryo is affected with this disease and to decide whether or not to proceed with the implantation. This is particularly important when it is known that one or both parents belong to the high-risk group.

Furthermore, PGD can be used to determine the child's sex or to identify genetically contingent characteristics. There are also documented cases in which the procedure was used to identify those embryos that were HLA-compatible with sick siblings so that the offspring could be available as a donor after the birth.

2.2. Various Ethical Assessments of PGD

From an ethical perspective, PGD is assessed in a number of different ways (see also Knoepffler 2004: 116–28; Kress 2003: 99–141; National Ethics Council 2003). Several standpoints can be differentiated. Various reasons are given for the complete rejection of PGD, but also for partial or complete acceptance of it, and some of these reasons are common to all.

One reason to reject all forms of PGD is contingent on the rejection of IVF, which is a necessary condition for PGD. In this case, IVF is considered immoral because it separates the progenitive act from the act of love, sexual intercourse (see also Catechism of the Catholic Church 1993: Number 2377). All forms of PGD can also be rejected independently of IVF, for example either when the totipotent cells are used up, meaning the cells from which a human being can develop, or because human embryos that are not implanted after a diagnosis are destroyed. Here, the embryos are granted the right to life. This would also apply if the passive euthanasia of newborns were possible (see below). Theoretically, there is additionally the possibility that diagnostics could serve a therapeutic function alone, which would mean that the embryos in question would be implanted in every case and, depending on the diagnostics, would undergo treatment as soon as possible. However, this theoretical possibility does not correspond to the current state in medicine. In practice, the use of PGD normally leads to the utilization of human beings in the earliest stages of development. Rejection of PGD is usually based on this fact. Furthermore, PGD is understood as a method of selection that, in the long run, could endanger human beings who have already been born and change our society for the worse.

Likewise, ethical assessments that consider PGD to be morally permissible are based on various arguments. Consequently, some accept only certain forms of PGD, while others would like to sanction all PGD procedures. Those who grant human embryos dignity and therefore consider PGD permissible only in situations in which non-implantation corresponds to passive euthanasia (see Knoepffler 2001) limit it to rare cases in which the embryos would die at the organogenesis (for example, Trisomy 15) or would have very short life expectancy (Trisomy 13 or 18, for example). Others want to extend the applicability of PGD to serious genetic diseases (see also German Association of MDs 2000) because they refer back to the unreasonable expectations of the parents, for example. Furthermore, there are others who argue that human embryos have not yet earned the right to protection. They consider other or even all forms of PGD morally permissible. This also includes PGD for gender selection, because they argue that parents have the right to decide which embryo should be implanted into the mother.

2.3. The Impossibility of Ethical Consensus as a Test Case for Tolerance

Arguments for ethical assessments of PGD show that ethical consensus is not possible. Those who reject IVF as immoral simply cannot consider any form of PGD acceptable. Those who grant dignity to embryos in the six- to ten-cell stage of development can agree to PGD only when it corresponds structurally to passive euthanasia. However, those who believe that a human embryo is not entitled to human dignity and that parents have a right to use the most modern technology with regard to their offspring will advocate PGD, in certain forms at any rate. Depending on the underlying moral options, advocates of PGD could even consider it morally reprehensible to deny parents this technology.

But why is consensus impossible? This will be explained with an example regarding the granting of human dignity. Those who are of the opinion that a six- to ten-celled embryo is deserving of dignity make a case for this with the species, continuity, identity or potentiality arguments. However, all of these arguments are controversial because the early development of an embryo can be morally interpreted in different ways. Before the fusion of genotypes of ovum and sperm, the early development does not show any significant defining moments (see also the discussion in Damschen and Schönecker 2002, and in Knoepffler 2004: 56–81). The argument that no person can be excluded from the legal community (Schweidler 2003) does not help much in this case because it is not exactly clear whether a human organism in the nascent stages of development is already a 'human being' or is still in a pre-stage of human existence. This can be demonstrated with a look at the situation at the end of life. In most cases, the end of a human being's life is equated with complete brain death. However, others disagree and advocate the thesis that the entire organism must be dead. In analogy to this, one could ask whether the beginning of human existence is present only when the neuronal structures first begin to develop – that is, after the formation of the primitive streak. Others disagree and argue for the zygote stage or even for the pronucleus stage. To avoid delving into this discussion, the following statement will suffice: at the moment, we are nowhere near the point at which ethical consensus is possible.

The legal discussion will not help us here either, even if we were to assume that we understand ethical consensus as an established law. The reason for this is very simple: at least in Germany, it is unclear whether embryos in a very early stage of development – that is, the point at which PGD is performed – have a right to human dignity according to current law. Therefore, it is not clear whether Article 1, Section 1 of the German Constitution, which states that human dignity is inviolable, refers also to human embryos. Moreover, both rulings of the German Constitutional Court 1975 and 1993 very plainly refer only to unborn embryos and foetuses from approximately the fourteenth day of development. For this reason the former Chief Justice of the German Constitutional Court, Jutta Limbach, stated very clearly:

> Both rulings do not enable one to make a prediction about how the Constitutional Court will rule on the legal status of an embryo produced in vitro because both decisions refer to traditional procreation. One can only guess how the Court will decide in the case of fertilization in the laboratory if it one day has to make a ruling about the constitutionality of pre-implantation diagnosis or therapeutic stem cell research on embryos produced in vitro that no longer have the potential to develop into a human being (Limbach, 2001).

Neither ethics nor the law can decide if PGD is permissible or not. How should the representatives of opposing, incompatible positions deal with one another? If we were to say that tolerance means that the opposing position is considered morally wrong, but not wrong in the sense that it would be impossible to at least (to a degree) tolerate the practices associated with it, then we are dealing with a test case for tolerance in this situation. Is it possible for opponents of PGD to be tolerant in this sense? Or, at the very least, is a condition for tolerance possible, namely that the opposing positions will be met with the necessary respect? In this context, respect means that one tries to have a fair-minded understanding of the other side and does not caricaturize it or defame it with misleading comparisons. Of course, respect does not mean that there cannot be good reasons for rejecting the position. Otherwise, one would not have to pose additional questions regarding whether the conflicting position can be 'tolerated'. When it is not tolerable, then the question takes on a socio-political dimension because it is now necessary to convey to the general public, though in a fair way, that such practice is not acceptable. It can also turn out that tolerance is the only way to reach a compromise that will serve society, at least on a political level. However, the kind of tolerance that allows room for the practices of the opposing side does not mean, of course, that these practices should be supported; on the contrary, in compromise situations it can be useful to define the breathing-room and for both sides to outline jointly a useful framework for tolerance. In contrast to a permission model of tolerance or a co-existence model of tolerance, this political respect model is characterized by the fact that the parties involved in the conflict respect each other as factions made up of moral subjects that each 'tolerate' the other. It is also shaped by the fact that a single resolution, which would entirely correspond to one's own convictions, cannot be found.

2.4. An Example of Intolerance

A counter-example will best demonstrate what was meant with regard to the concept of tolerance developed within the framework of PGD. This example is very important, as in a certain way it shows how far we are from this point in Germany both individually, because the prerequisite of mutual interaction, which states that the opinions of others need to be respected, is being violated, and politically, because one evades the respect model in human biotechnological conflict situations that are ethically and legally controversial. For this reason, the example has not been taken from just any publication, but rather from the report 'The Constitutional Status of Embryos in vitro' of the Enquête Commission of the German Parliament, 'Legal and Ethical Issues of Modern Medicine'. On the one hand, this report has an individualized dimension as the opinion of an expert, and on the other hand it has a political dimension as a report for the German Parliament. The text reads as follows:

> Assuming that the decision regarding whether or not one can be born was parallel to pre-implantation diagnosis, then the similarities to the worst crimes of the Nazi regime would be obvious. It is about a decision to deny a person the right to live because of certain characteristics. The image of the selection ramp in Auschwitz unavoidably comes to mind in the same way as a 'euthanasia programme' directed at handicapped persons. The decision regarding whether or not someone's life is 'worthy' or 'unworthy' is left up to others who enforce their judgement in action; that is, in the ending of 'unworthy' lives. An even more forceful basic questioning of the 'human as subject' is unthinkable (Sacksofsky 2001: 47).

The conditional 'assuming' seems to represent an attenuation. In relation to the entire report, however, this conditional allegation is incomprehensible because of consistency problems and is, therefore, a clear sign of disrespect towards advocates of PGD. Why is this allegation inconsistent? It is not consistent because in another section the following emerges:

> A concept in which the protection of life gradually increases is more justified than the categorical postulate that a fertilized ovum is to be equally treated as a human being because it reflects the development of an embryo. The public debate over the permissibility of genetic research is based on a fundamental schism of opinions. While one side sees a fertilized ovum as nothing more than an 'accumulation of cells', the other side considers a fertilized ovum to be a whole human being. The concept in which the protection of life gradually increases successfully combines both points of view. The fertilized ovum is simultaneously an 'accumulation of cells' and a 'person in progress'. Because a fertilized ovum is also a 'person in progress', it cannot be treated as raw material or an object; translated into legal language, this means: it is to be granted the constitutional right to protection of life. On the other hand, because a fertilized ovum is fundamentally different than a (completed) human being, it has less right to protection than a human being who has already been born. The fertilized ovum can develop into a completed human being, but it is not one yet (Sacksofsky 2001: 27).

For this reason, the central point of the latter passage is disputed. What is the point of having this reference to National Socialism if it is acknowledged that a fertilized ovum can be fundamentally differentiated from a (completed) human being, which is why it has less right to the protection of life as that of a human being who has already been born? In this case, it is not possible to grant it the quality of 'human as subject'. Following up on the last quoted passage, it appears particularly grotesque in the subsequent statement:

> With the aid of such an interpretation, consistent answers to problem constellations become possible, which absolutizing points of view cannot afford' (Sacksofsky 2001: 27).

With regard to PGD, the following sums it up:

> As a result, pre-implantation diagnosis violates both the right to human dignity and an in vitro embryo's basic right to the freedom from bodily harm as well as the objective dimension of the principle of human dignity. In this respect, legislators do not have any elbowroom. Pre-implantation diagnosis must be and remain banned (Sacksofsky 2001: 27).

Even if we do not follow the report's inconsistency, but rather advocate a position in which a human embryo is considered to be a human being in a moral sense, then the comparison with the crimes of National Socialism and the example of an intolerant attitude, in the sense that the respect of the opinions of others is violated, remain untenable. On the one hand, there is the possibility to use PGD on pluripotent cells in order to avoid implanting embryos that, to some degree, are already in the process of dying, whether it be during organogenesis or shortly after birth. This inaction is comparable to passive euthanasia because it is current medical practice to forego maximum medical care and to allow passive euthanasia when the newborns are already in the process of dying, and it is what the parents want. It is then out of the question that in such instances either human dignity or the right to freedom from bodily harm are violated. Comparing this form of PGD with Nazi crimes is completely absurd.

Furthermore, the comparison is inapplicable because all forms of PGD that are presently being discussed as political options represent the decisions of individuals, which means that it is in no way a government programme in which the decisions are dictated from the top down. There is no differentiation made between the killing of human organisms against the will of those concerned or the inaction at the request of the parents when one believes that these organisms have no will and are neither persons nor subjects according to the advocates of PGD. Even for supporters of PGD, the issue is not about choosing between 'worthy' and 'unworthy' lives because they do not consider the embryos to be human beings that are not going to be implanted; rather, they are a pre-form of human existence.

Even if we were to assume that such a government programme existed that would demand a PGD and even if we were to consider a human embryo to be both a person and a subject, the comparison with Nazi crimes remains doubly disrespectful to the Holocaust. On the one hand, the unimaginable crimes against the Jews motivated by racial mania and conspiracy theories, for which the term 'Auschwitz' now stands, would be instrumentalized in order to put a rejected position in the worst possible light. This is even more objectionable for the fact that one indirectly links present-day Israel, where PGD is legal, with the crimes of National Socialism. At the same time, supporters of PGD are associated with the criminal Nazi regime. We should also remember that we now honour those who wanted to kill the leader of this criminal regime as heroes of conscience. Put very bluntly, should advocates of PGD be treated in the same way as those responsible for the crimes at Auschwitz, who, like Eichmann, were sentenced to death? In connection with this, we must keep in mind that within the abortion debate those who opposed abortion did indeed kill doctors who performed them and in a similar way referred to their right to protect the unborn in need from what they considered criminal actions.

Of course, we should not presume that the author would like similar consequences in relation to PGD. Rather, it should now be clear how quickly a bioethical conflict can extend into a sort of religious war that labels those who think differently as criminals. And do not those who reject religious freedom have good reasons when considered within the context of the passage quoted in section 2.3? Are those people who prevent their children from being 'saved' (as a result of poor upbringing) worse than someone who kills a human embryo? Does this justify a restriction on religious freedom and maybe even the persecution of heretics as a form of assistance for people with weak determination or even a religious war as a form of help on a grand scale? At least in the Western world, the great accomplishment of the last century was the recognition (as the result of difficult experiences with religious war) that this kind of war is no solution to conflict and that a ban on religious freedom represents the wrong approach. At the very least, the major Christian denominations have taken the hard road in order to take small steps towards each other, to try to understand each other a little bit better and to see the commonalities, rather than the differences, between them. In this way, for example, in 1965 the Roman Catholic and the Orthodox Catholic Churches were able to erase the letters of excommunication from 1054 from their memories. And in Augsburg, Germany in 1999, the Roman

Catholic and Lutheran Churches decided that the two-way denunciations relative to Luther's justification theology no longer applied to contemporary viewpoints.

3. Conditions for a Culture of Tolerance in Bioethical Debates

A few of the conditions for a culture of respect and tolerance in bioethical debates have been identified within this context. Moreover, a culture of tolerance could replace the current bioethical 'battle of the cultures' (Kreß 2004: 39).

The first fundamental condition requires that each side clearly and consistently present its argument. It is not a matter of abandoning one's own convictions, but rather giving one's own opinion with the best possible argument. For example, in the PGD debate, the point is not to grant human embryos in the six- to ten-celled stage the right to human dignity in the sense of principle equality and principle status as subject. Along these same lines, in the abortion debate the point is not that human embryos that have a beating heart and human face are not to be understood as human beings with regard to principle equality and principle status as subject because of gradually increasing protection of life; or in other words, to deprive them of human dignity. Indeed, the reverse would be inconsistent. There are certainly enough reasons not to consider an embryo to be a human being already that has a right to human dignity. This is true, for example, when we assume that a human embryo is not yet an individual in the strict sense of the word and therefore does not yet live as a human being because it does not yet exhibit neuronal activities. However, at the same time it is possible to hold the opinion that an embryo that already has a human face and exhibits the first neuronal activity has a right to human dignity and is to be treated, in principle, as an equal and subject. Likewise, there are consistent positions that regard PGD and abortion as morally permissible as well as other consistent positions that reject both PGD and abortion. Of course, the arguments for all of these positions can be questioned for reasons that should be taken seriously.

The second condition is: keeping respect for others in mind, challenging of other positions needs to be done without all forms of defamation. For example, defamation could have a structure that assumes that representatives of other opinions have unfair or base motives. Ernst-Ludwig Winnacker, the president of the German Research Foundation, must have experienced this when he lobbied for embryonic stem cell research in 2001. He was accused of wanting to enhance his own financial situation through stem cell research and being ready to sacrifice his 'ethical' principles for it. However, defamation can take on another form, namely that those who have other opinions will be presumed to be fundamentalists or irrational. Such presumptions are made in place of carefully examining the other position. Pope John Paul II likely experienced this when he prohibited the Roman Catholic Church in Germany from counselling pregnant women about abortion. Moreover, respect as a precondition for tolerance requires that the arguments of the opposing side be benevolent and not be examined malevolently. The guiding principle should then be dependent on the classic sixteenth-century idea of Ignatius Loyola, which declares that arguments of the opposing side should be salvaged when possible and not condemned. When they can no longer be salvaged, then one needs to ask whether the argument was truly understood. And this is respectful even in a case where repudiation is necessary (see also Ignatius Loyola 1988: No. 22).

Furthermore, having respect for representatives of other points of view does not demand that we must forego advocating our own position under the rules of the majority. This kind of promotion should, however, not be qualified as immoral by supporters of the opposing position. This kind of respect can lead to respectful tolerance and render willingness to compromise possible with regard to conflicts that are argumentatively no longer resolvable on a societal level, for example when we are dealing with political decisions. A compromise relative to the PGD test case could turn out like this, meaning that these procedures are, for example, not covered by medical insurance and that only certain objectives are permitted. A good compromise should avoid ethical and legal inconsistencies, as seen in the rulings of the German Constitutional Court with regard to abortion (after Merkel 2002: 65):

- If a woman can provide proof of family planning counselling, then a contract for abortion agreed upon by the doctor and pregnant woman is effective despite the fact that abortion is called an unlawful killing of a person with legal rights in paragraphs 134 and 138 of the German Civil Law Book (*Bundesgesetzbuch*).
- All emergency assistance for the benefit of the unborn whose subjective right to life is violated and who, according to the ruling of the German Constitutional Court, has a right to human dignity is not permitted.
- A woman who seeks an abortion may claim sick pay for the time required for the unlawful act of killing.
- The government is obliged to guarantee 'adequate and nationwide opportunities for abortions and both outpatient and inpatient facilities' (German Constitutional Court 88, 328f.).

The point here is not to make straightforward recommendations for individual conflict situations in the bioethical domain. It should merely be pointed out that without having to abandon one's own beliefs there is the possibility that these recommendations can be introduced into a respectful dialogue between representatives of diverse standpoints and political compromises can perhaps be found. And these compromises show that we do not have to accept the other position, but may 'put up with it' and tolerate legal elbowroom for opposing points of view. Compromises that have already been made relative to the exemption from punishment for the abetment of suicide, the acquisition of prophylactics and the 'abortion' pill and divorce laws are examples of a culture of respect and tolerance. Moreover, there are almost no public protests or demonstrations within this scope. Those who reject these regulations, for example because they reject suicide and all forms of assisted suicide, or believe that contraceptives such as the pill are immoral, or consider marriage to be indissoluble, nevertheless respectfully tolerate the predominating regulations. This kind of respectful tolerance does not have to go so far that we must adopt it. In this way, a Roman Catholic employer can terminate the employment contract of a pre-school teacher who re-marries, but no active steps are taken to make it difficult for her to find a job in a public pre-school. In this case, the Roman Catholic Church respectfully tolerates the governmental regulations, though they do not correspond to Church regulations. The Church also explicitly allows Roman Catholic politicians to assist in finding compromises that do not correspond to the teachings of the Catholic Church if even greater injury can be avoided (John Paul II 1995: No. 73). Thereby, the Church allows respect and tolerance on a political level.

For these reasons, the hope exists that we can find solutions to bioethical conflict situations such as PGD and active euthanasia that are compatible with society and can at the very least be tolerated by all sides.

Bibliography

Bundesärztekammer [German Association of MDs] (2000) 'Diskussionsentwurf zu einer Richtlinie zur Präimplantationsdiagnostik', *Deutsches Ärzteblatt*, **97**, C-423–C-426

Catechism of the Catholic Church (1993) München: Oldenbourg

Claussen, U. (2001) 'Präimplantationsdiagnostik (PID) – Eine kritische Stellungnahme', *Ärzteblatt Thüringen*, **12**, 392–8

Damschen, G., and **Schönecker, D.** (eds) (2002) *Der moralische Status menschlicher Embryonen – Pro und contra Spezies-, Kontinuums-, Identitäts- und Potentialitätsargument*, Berlin: Walter de Gruyter Books

Forst, R. (2003) *Toleranz im Konflikt – Geschichte, Gehalt und Gegenwart eines umstrittenen Begriffs*, Frankfurt am Main: Suhrkamp

Ignatius von Loyola (1988) *Geistliche Übungen und erläuternde Texte*, third edn, Graz: Styria

John Paul II (1995) *Evangelium Vitae*, *fourth edn* (ed. Secretariat of the German Bishops' Conference), Bonn: (ohne Verlag)

Knoepffler, N. (2001) 'Nicht-Implantation des Embryos nach Präimplantationsdiagnostik (PGD) als passive Sterbehilfe in bestimmbaren Fällen', *Medizinische Genetik*, **13**, 305–8

Knoepffler, N. (2004) *Menschenwürde in der Bioethik*, Berlin: Springer Publishing

Kreß, H. (2003) *Medizinische Ethik – Kulturelle Grundlagen und ethische Wertkonflikte heutiger Medizin*, Stuttgart: Kohlhammer

Kreß, H. (2004) 'Religionsfreiheit und Toleranz als Leitbild – Kulturelle Grundlagen – Sozial- und rechtsethische Problemstellungen', in Kreß (ed.), *Religionsfreiheit Als Leitbild – Staatskirchenrecht in Deutschland und Europa im Prozess der Reform*, Münster: LIT, 21–58

Limbach, J. (2001) 'Menschenwürde und medizinischer Fortschritt', at www.medizinundgewissen.de/limbachrede.html, accessed on 15 February 2005

Merkel, R. (2002) *Forschungsobjekt Embryo – Verfassungsrechtliche und ethische Grundlagen der Forschung an menschlichen embryonalen Stammzellen*, München: Dtv

Nationaler Ethikrat [National Ethics Council] (2003) Genetische Diagnostik vor und während der Schwangerschaft – Stellungnahme, Berlin: (ohne Verlag)

Sacksofsky, U. (2001) *Der Verfassungsrechtliche Status des Embryos in vitro Gutachten für die Enquete-Kommission des Deutschen Bundestages 'Recht und Ethik der modernen Medizin'*, Frankfurt am Main: (ohne Verlag)

Schweidler, W. (2003) 'Zur Analogie des Lebensbegriffs und ihrer bioethischen Relevanz', in Schweidler (ed.), *Menschenleben – Menschenwürde. Interdisziplinäres Symposium zur Bioethik*, Münster: LIT, 13–29

Chapter Ten

Human Biotechnology as an Ethical and Social Challenge

Julian Nida-Rümelin

I would like to begin with two prefaces. First, I find very interesting the way that the organizers planned the opening of this conference, namely with two lectures that address the empirical dimensions of what we are here to discuss. Recently, at the European Academy in Bad Neuenahr, I proposed that philosophical ethics needs the support of empiricism.[1] Second, as was mentioned in those kind words of introduction, from 1991 to 2003 I was Professor for 'Ethics in Life Sciences', an endowed professorship in Baden-Württemberg, which is now an established chair currently occupied by my successor, Eva-Marie Engels. This position presented me with the fascinating opportunity to head a centre for ethics in the sciences, which brought together seven departments each contributing their particular disciplinary perspectives. Among other issues, we debated intensely the ethical questions of genetic engineering. It was a constant struggle merely to find a common language or at least to develop a sufficiently broad overlap in the languages of our different disciplines in order to make sound communication possible.

The following is a perfect example of the widespread misunderstanding amid the struggle for clear communication. A few days before the beginning of my appointment as National Minister of Culture, I was asked by the Culture Editor of *Tagesspiegel* (a national left-leaning newspaper) to succinctly explain my position on the decision of the British Parliament to allow therapeutic cloning before an embryo implants itself in the mother's womb. I explained that the British model ought not to be adopted in Germany at this time, even though there was no fundamental or absolute ethical objection to the British decision. This position would hardly have appeared scandalous but for *Tagesspiegel*'s treatment of it with a page one article under the bright red headline, 'Nida-Rümelin: Human cloning, why not?'[2] Such are the ignoble ways in which misunderstanding can affect our public discourse, particularly when strong political interests are at play.

And with that I arrive at the actual topic of my lecture, which I want to address in three ways. First of all, I shall address the question regarding what role ethics plays and what philosophy as a discipline can accomplish. Second, I shall ask what

---

1 This refers to the Spring Conference of the European Academy concerned with the consequences of scientific and technological developments, from 31 March to 2 April 2004. The conference theme was 'The Interdisciplinary Function of Philosophy.'

2 The article and subsequent discussion are documented in my (2002) *Ethical Essays*, part IV, Frankfurt am Main: Suhrkamp.

the social and moral–ethical challenges to the new biotechnologies are. And third, I want to present a few arguments regarding the subject matter; a statement about my position, so to speak.

First of all, what role does ethics play? It seems to me that a rather strange situation has developed in answer to this question. On the one hand, there is the common expectation that philosophy – and, in particular, ethics – can and does give us direction with regard to practical matters. On the other hand, ethics is relegated to a minor role in the public discourse, namely in the form of meaningless words, and should be kept out of the research process. For example, this is reflected in Germany's many ethics commissions made up primarily of theologians or jurists who have practically no philosophical expertise. The situation is very different in the US.

To take a step back from the matter at hand, I think that our lives – whether in research, in the everyday, or in intimate social relations – are shaped almost completely by our values. One example is the value of *respect for personal autonomy*, a humanistic orientation central to a free society, which says each person is responsible for his or her own life. Therefore, there are probably good reasons for what he or she wants and does, and I may not interfere even if I think I know better what is good for someone else. *Personal autonomy* in conjunction with Articles 1 to 19 of the German Constitution is not only the basis of jurisprudence, but also shapes our daily activities, research policies and the ways that we *deal* with medical innovation. In this way, a fundamental change in modern medicine is taking place, which is moving away from the ethics of paternalism. Paternalism implies that the physician knows what is best for the patient and accordingly makes the decisions while the patient gladly accepts them and subordinates to the physician. Instead, we now have the ethics of 'informed consent', a term used also in Germany. This means that there is concurrence between the one being treated, the patient, and the one treating, the physician. The patient, having been well informed by the physician, decides which treatment he or she wants.

However, if our social lives are impregnated by moral values, standards and rules, what, if anything, can theoretical reflection and ethics contribute? Are not the most important aspects already fixed through the codification of certain core elements of these moral orientations? For example, from an ethical standpoint, do we need more than Article 1 of the Constitution and everything that is based upon it? My answer is yes and no. I stand in opposition to most ethicists of the twentieth century when I say that ethics cannot specify an Archimedean point from which we can derive what is ethically right and wrong. Neither Kant's Categorical Imperative nor some utilitarian principle can serve as such an Archimedean point. Of late, that was also a problem of the 'Singer debate'. Peter Singer and many others who also advocate a utilitarian approach believe they have a rationally grounded principle that with the help of empirical observation will assist us in recognizing what is right and wrong. But that is not how it works, because when there are serious contradictions between the deductions of an ethical theory and those of certain secular moral intuitions, theory typically loses.

Nevertheless, ethical theory can accomplish the following: it can point out where there are incoherencies and contradictions in those supposedly irrefutable secular, moral convictions. Thus, rules that are usually accepted as self-evident cannot always be absolutely maintained. Doubt first sets in when one thing becomes clear: aha, something is not right with what I think is right. At this point, demand for reflection and ethical clarity arises. This is precisely the task of philosophy.

I am convinced that a *coherent basis* is not just one basis among many, but rather one without alternative. Philosophy and, in principle, science can only proceed coherently. With that being the case, it is not a matter of deciding between ethical criteria on the one hand and economic criteria on the other, because there are no genuine conflicts between ethics and economics, even if some would like to think so. The fundamental question is always, what actions and activities are correct and justifiable? In answering this question, 'good' ethics must include economic as well as scientific elements in its argumentation.

Naturally, there are some differences in worldviews that rational argument cannot resolve. And considering the very difficult question of how to deal with new technologies, it would be quite illusory to hope that we could set aside fundamental differences through rational argument. This has already turned out to be hopeless in the abortion debate and now even more so with regard to the biotechnology debate. The important question is, how does a society deal with perpetually irresolvable differences in worldviews? An example of one difference is that some say human dignity makes absolutely no sense unless interpreted theologically as an expression of mankind's creation in God's image. Others say they simply do not share the same religion or religious conviction, but agree with Kant that human dignity provides an important normative orientation. These two factions will not be able to come to an agreement about the basis of human dignity. However, there is common ground. For example, it may be possible to communicate through what John Rawls calls a normative 'overlapping consensus', despite continued differences in worldviews. And that is precisely what makes a deliberative democracy deliberative: it offers solutions based on this common ground that seem acceptable to people with different worldviews. The ultimate foundation for values will be seen as different, but understanding is made possible. I believe that this is the direction in which we should steer the biotechnology debate.

I come now to my second point: what exactly are the ethical and social challenges created by the new biotechnology? I shall now name four facets. First, since the European Enlightenment or actually since the emergence of fourteenth-century Italian Humanism, we have had a strong normative orientation towards learning and self-directed education based on the idea that a person *qua* person need not remain as nature or social status has formed him or her. Rather, people can self-evolve beyond their natural and social limitations. In connection with this, language and interaction with other cultures played a central role, and they continue to do so. The essence of the idea of learning and self-directed education is fundamental to our contemporary self-image. For example, even today we try to create the most favourable educational and learning conditions for ourselves and for later generations. Incidentally, I mean education and learning not in the narrow sense of 'schooling'. Our descendants should be allowed to freely develop beyond their limits, as should we. Nevertheless, this concept of education encompasses certain limitations: one can develop and improve, but there are things we cannot change, for example congenital diseases or the overall physical composition of humans, because we have no influence over them. At present, it appears completely unrealistic that the new biotechnology will be able to alter our genetic code substantially. One day in the future, it will probably be used to cure some congenital diseases, but essentially little will change for decades; the arguments for this conclusion have already been mentioned by both scientists who spoke previously. Nonetheless, this 'science fiction' dimension of biotechnology occupies people's imaginations. This is logical and understandable, especially considering the early days of genetic research in the 1950s and 1960s when scientists spun hopeful fantasies to drum up public and financial support for their projects.

Second, there is conflict between the tendency towards ever wider distinctions in experts' qualifications, on the one hand, and an ever greater call for responsible safeguards, on the other. It is completely unthinkable to delegate ethical responsibility for biotechnology to a single authority such as a political or legislative body. Rather, we need people, including those who are doing the research, to bring an ethical sensibility and corresponding responsibility to help create actively the field of ethical responsibility. The coupling of science with competence in the humanities is urgently necessary and should not be a superfluous, but rather an integral educational component, particularly regarding ethical competence in science education. The Ethics Centre in Tübingen is an attempt in this direction, in its constructive attempts to link expertise with responsibility.

Third, morality does not result from reflection alone but, according to Aristotelians, it comes about, to a large extent, from experience, habit and traditions that are handed down from one generation to the next. It is misleading to think that it is possible to conjure up a new ethos that people will readily accept as generally binding simply by means of rationalistic gesture. The quicker the societal, scientific, technological and international situation changes, the stronger the pressure for an established ethos to change becomes. In an enlightened society, these processes of change will be accompanied by public discourse that walks us not only through reflective arguments, but also through various interest-driven viewpoints, for example political or economic. It can be extremely difficult to pursue arguments in the face of deep-seated interests, and I worry that, in the genetic engineering debate, the agenda for public discourse will be set by well-established interests that make reasonable communication all the more difficult. This plays out, for example, in the National Ethics Advisory Council, which is composed of a unique combination of interdisciplinary experts, on the one hand, and special interest group spokespersons, on the other. You can sense here the German political coalition tradition at work, but at the same time this presents a danger for rational discourse. The spokesperson of a certain interest group is duty-bound to the views of the group and, should the occasion arise, is inclined to simply ignore other arguments.

Fourth, we are accustomed to extending our moral judgements to things that we have under control or things we can foresee. Hans Jonas once called this 'short-sighted ethics'. The new technologies in general and in biotechnology in particular now compel us towards a *far-sighted ethics* because the consequences of new technologies are so complex, and their long-term effects are difficult to assess. Moral judgement has a hard time with these issues because the question of how we handle new technology demands that ethics integrate a great deal of empiricism. That in itself is foreign to the ethical tradition. It is distressing for me to see this empirical element, which earlier was included in the category of the assessment of the effects of technology, now being largely marginalized by it. In order to develop a balanced legal solution to these long-term scenarios and perspectives, I think we must once again try to bring empirical scientific and sociological knowledge together with knowledge from the humanities. I call this approach *values holism*.

In closing, I would like to attempt to sketch out a few subject-orientated positions. The first important aspect is the *gradualistic* interpretation in which 'becoming human' is a continuous process. Still, boundaries must be set in ethics and in law. For example, in Germany one must be at least 18 years of age to drive a car. That is ultimately an arbitrary choice, but since we would like to have secure and clear boundaries for driving permits or voting rights these albeit arbitrary boundaries are legitimate. This applies to many continuous processes, for example coming of age. Of course, there are some unmistakable turning points in these processes, particularly in the area of biology. The implantation or nidation of a foetus is one such turning point; in my opinion, the moment of totipotence is even more significant. This is a decisive phase inasmuch as it is distinguished from later phases of the human foetus since one cannot logically hold that there is a relationship of identity between the early-phase inseminated egg cell and the fully developed individual. This would break the transitive character of identity: if A is identical to B and B is to C, then A is identical to C. Christian ethics with its dogmatic attribution of human dignity at the moment of insemination of the ovum is simply based on erroneous empirical assumptions. Still, there are important Christian ethicists in the German-speaking world who use arguments for gradualism similar to mine, such as the Protestant theologian Richard Schröder and the Jesuit priest Christian Kummer.

In my opening remarks, I indicated that coherence and the scrutinizing of coherence are the essential tasks of philosophy. Of course, it is true that there can be completely different opinions concerning the fundamental issue of suitable criteria for ascribing human dignity. However, it is necessary that every opinion be coherent with other opinions we have. It is not possible for us to accept particular models of behaviour and particular legal rules and regulations that rest unambiguously on a gradualist ethic, while at the same time say that none of it applies to biotechnology. The following is an example of a flagrant contradiction: the ethical evaluation of the IUD as contraceptive – which is to say, the prevention of the nesting of the inseminated egg – in comparison with the dogmatic ascription of human dignity to the inseminated egg before its nesting. These two ethical evaluations cannot co-exist because those who are convinced that the foetus deserves full rights to human dignity from the day of insemination could not consider this form of contraception harmless. They would have to support punitive consequences for this practice, not to mention for the applicable abortion laws. To those who hold such a 'fundamentalist' position, I should ask that they bear in mind the dangers connected with such fundamentalism for the normative efficacy of the notion of human dignity. I myself attempt to strengthen the human dignity argument by limiting the concept to the essence of its application. We ought not to endanger this normative fundamentalist consensus that influences not only our constitution but also our everyday social interactions.[3]

The second important aspect concerns the question of *responsibility*, which is particularly urgent when it comes to biotechnology. A society like ours, which is based on humanistic individualism, must also hold the principle of personal responsibility in high regard. Naturally, there are limits, for example, wherever others could be injured by the inappropriate exercise of personal responsibility. In any case, the essential function of law is to fix and secure these limits. But within these limits, responsibility can and must be taken by the individual and taken very seriously in cases such as parents who are faced with the new biotechnology.

The third aspect concerns conflicts of values that we admittedly cannot address because they are dependent to some extent on considerable differences in worldviews. But it is precisely because of these differences that the process of consensus-building leads us to a common ground. We are just at the beginning, but I am convinced that education has to accept a larger role in this process. Shortening the length of time spent in school and university seems like a good idea, but the accompanying tendency towards the *instrumentalization* of education in terms of 'preparation for…' is counterproductive. Even current labour market developments, which claim that the best preparation for career training comes from a solid education, would disagree with this tendency. The better the educational background, the easier it is, in most occupations, to orientate oneself and continue to learn, change jobs, deal with other cultures, and so on. To be qualified for only one narrow occupational specialization appears to be neither sensible nor efficient. The necessary changes to our education system must keep in mind more specifically that education is not only about preparation, but also about good old-fashioned character-building. *Character-building* means the ability to make judgements and act responsibly. It also means struggling and coming to terms with differences, handling contradictions among value systems, and attempting to find an acceptable compromise on common ground. It is impossible simply to delegate this process to philosophy or ethics, or to theology or politics. It can function only as a process in which the entire society takes part and in which each contributes his or her expertise as scientist, as philosopher, as jurist, and so on. Likewise, all participants must act responsibly. For example, each must resist the temptation to exploit the process of consensus for a political sideshow or ideological skirmishing. In particular, we have to be careful not to make difficult questions appear easily resolvable by falling back on moral taboo according to which we all supposedly know from the outset the moral right and wrong; for example, that it is morally unacceptable to interfere with the human germination process. We must avoid unconditionally such regression and uphold the process as well as the results of rational clarification. The same goes for the prohibition against human embryonic pre-implantation diagnostics in Germany. Why this prohibition is presented as a perfectly reasonable, unquestionably valid moral principle is difficult to comprehend. The arguments for and against a ban must be discussed rationally

3 Cf. my 'Human Dignity and Self Respect', in *Self Respect or Self Acceptance? Contributions toward a Theory of Justice and Human Dignity*, in the series *Writings of the Friedrich Nietzsche Colloquium*, Weimar.

and a solution, legal and ethical, must be found on the common ground discussed above.

I would like to close with the observation that we cannot avoid the process of clarification and consensus-building when dealing with the new biotechnology. We cannot simply say, 'Let's just clarify that for now, and then we can let science do its thing.' Naturally, this process is tiring, especially with its enormous public attention, countless debates, and sometimes enlightening yet often completely pointless and terribly misleading newspaper articles. But we have to walk this road together, because it concerns the fundamentals of our self-understanding as scientists, as private individuals, and as members of this democratically structured society.

Chapter Eleven

Bioethics between *Physis* and *Nomos*

Gianni Vattimo

Is it possible to find criteria and boundaries for assessing the morality of our decisions within the concept of 'human nature'? This is a question that has become increasingly urgent, though at the same time it is often demonized in a world in which modern technoscience has brought about many changes in our lives. Even if one is intimately familiar with critical modern thought and its historicist implications, one feels drawn (though we could also say tempted) to return to the notion of a natural set of rules; a notion that critical thinkers of the last two centuries (from Marx to Nietzsche, from Freud to Adorno) taught us to mistrust. Too many times what has been passed off as 'human nature' in the form of this or that doctrine is actually just an ideal of humanity that corresponds to certain social conditions or, in a positive sense, to certain contingent interests. For example, if it is necessary to go to war, then we say, 'Be a man!', which implies that 'man', according to his nature, must be ready to go to war.

Yet, when one reflects about issues in the vein of gene manipulation, but also more 'traditional' ones such as abortion, nature seems to come back into the picture. Should embryos be granted respect because human beings have dignity at the very moment of their conception? Or should they have dignity merely because they will be able to make decisions for themselves someday? (In the latter case, do we then have the right to kill human beings who will not become subjects of freedom and following from that subjects deserving human dignity because of some serious handicap?) Recently, a number of cases similar to the following example have emerged: a French citizen, born with too many physical handicaps to live a normal life, took legal action against the public health system for not having helped his mother to abort.

Even before the technical possibility of prenatal diagnosis, it was well known that the 'natural' birth of a person was actually not all that natural, because the decision to have a child was made wilfully. It has been like this for generations, even in cases of unwanted children. However, no child has yet taken action against his or her parents because they were either unmarried or poor, or were born in less than ideal social or political conditions, or had a serious genetic disease. Up to what point are parents responsible for the genetic endowment of their children? Should a mother who smokes or an alcoholic father be legally prosecuted and perhaps be obliged to indemnify the child for the damages caused by the parents' lifestyle? These are just some extreme examples to better explain the problem.

Recently, Jürgen Habermas, the last great representative of the Frankfurt School, considered this matter. In a recent book, Habermas calls attention to the term 'human nature', which, if we understand correctly, was not that central in his previous writings, in which he discussed, for example, the conditions of a 'good life'. These conditions are more or less identified (to quote Alastair McIntyre) with those in which everyone is free to decide for himself what the good life is. This is a position that shapes the criteria for the good life based on the idea of freedom together with concepts of history and culture, while not focusing too much on biological aspects, which could be used as arguments against abortion. In his latest work, which focuses on genetic manipulation, Habermas proposes an Aristotelian attitude, which distinguishes between the spontaneous and the artificial – the *Gewachsene* and the *Gemachte*. In other words, it is the difference between that which grows and that which is made. The difference in Aristotle's writings is clear, but not really that precise: *technê* in many cases finishes what nature does not, even if it could (for example, cooking is a way of anticipating the natural digestion process), and in other cases does what nature cannot do. Also in these cases, artists and technicians respect some natural 'rule', which has nothing to do with the objectively endowed traits of a living thing. Their set of rules is certainly 'human nature' – but it does not refer to what a human being, as a natural being, is, or what he would become if he were to let 'nature' take over. Let us also remember that, according to Aristotle's *Ethics*, in order to find out whether a man is virtuous, we must ask others in his community. This is clearly a more historical and cultural criterion than a 'natural' one. With regard to human 'nature', it is likely that Aristotle never adopted a fiercely essentialist point of view. In this sense, the limits we find in 'nature' are nothing but rigid metaphysical notions.

What about genetic manipulation? In a recent interview for *Le Monde*, Habermas said that if parents were to manipulate their son's genes during his development, in order to make of him a great musician like Beethoven, this would be a violation of his freedom, because maybe he really wanted to become a pilot. The problem is, what is either natural or spontaneous about his desire to become a great pilot? Did his mother watch too many movies about aviation when she was pregnant?

In conclusion, does human nature develop independently, whose only condition is that two people of different sexes came together to make a baby (either using or not using a condom, or waiting to have a flat of their own or a job, and so on)? Maybe we should mention not just Aristotle, but also Pico della Mirandola, who determined the nature of man in the very fact that he does not have a nature or a definite essence, and must shape himself.

Keeping all of this in mind and turning to law, it is not possible to reduce the whole matter to the distinction between what is 'grown' and what is 'made' (produced); in fact, man produces spontaneously and does not always let nature takes its course. However, Habermas fears the excesses of a liberal attitude towards genetics; in other words, manipulation without limits and influenced by market interests. He goes on to ask what human beings will feel in the future having been born via all kinds of technological manipulations. How does a robot feel knowing that it is a robot? We obviously shudder when we look at the situation in such a way. But ultimately the boundary that we must set cannot be metaphysical or universal (for example, recently democracy has sometimes been imposed on countries through violence), but instead it must be historical. It is something 'natural', meaning that which appears to be natural under certain conditions of existence. Using a simple example, it is 'natural' to say hello to someone walking down the street, even if no metaphysical law imposes it on us. Laws can only be based on this 'natural' criterion if they have to fit into a democratic political order. For example, abortion is currently legal in many countries, but doctors have the freedom of conscientious objection. Many pro-lifers consider this to go beyond the law of nature. But, again, the dangers of comparing democracy-based parliamentary decisions with allegedly 'natural laws' are very clear (they amount to what is called an 'ethical state'). For this reason, the only naturally human way at our disposal is to accept the freedom of conscience as a rule. A nation is not an ethical subject, in the same sense that it is not an aesthetic, religious or theoretical one. There is no scientific truth officially adopted by the state, no religion, no style of art, and so on. Interpreting the notion of 'nature' and of 'natural' in the sense I just proposed, is simply a reaction to the demands of a modern democracy, which is undoubtedly based on the belief that we have a natural right to freedom and to shared societal decisions, but does not involve, or cannot involve, any communal belief in an essential structure of reality, of human nature, and so on. In many ways, freedom is not a 'truth' which a democratic state should recognize as such, but rather it is just a practical means by which the people can limit the power of persons in power. It seems to me that in relation also to the 'extreme' questions created by today's biology and biotechnology, the sole rationality we can accept as a norm is the reasonability of our shared opinions. It is probably not an historical coincidence that democratic societies have developed alongside what can only be called 'nihilism' or 'the end of metaphysics', using Heidegger's words. Regardless of which is the cause and which the effect, the fact is that our society is principally founded upon democratic structures and, at the same time, no longer has strong metaphysical certitudes. Any appeal to a basic undeniable truth about the 'nature' – of man, of family or of life itself – sounds like an attempt to restore authoritarianism.

We are all aware of the grave seriousness of the questions with which we are faced in the field of bioethics. But this does not give us the right to return to a pre-modern, pre-liberal or even pre-Christian way of dealing with an individual's right to freedom. Identifying God's will with that which occurs 'spontaneously' in nature is just a remnant of ancient superstitions. I think it is also a case of suspicion against any form of human genetic manipulation. Let me repeat that I am fully aware of the seriousness of the questions with which we are confronted. In my opinion, however, the only 'human' way of dealing with them is to establish a set of regulations for the entire domain that is based on explicit negotiations that are free from all dogmatic and metaphysical assumptions. What is extraordinary is the fact that we have been thrown into a world in which human genes can be manipulated. (Nietzsche would say that we have the ability to freely determine our 'natural' constitution, and that we should raise ourselves to the level of this new ability.) Up until now, this was our fate and we could only accept it. There is no ethical or religious reason for us to refuse to accept this natural responsibility.

If we consider the responsibility of individuals and of society in light of these problems, it is just the first step towards finding a democratic solution. Simply put, if there was a natural rule that had been respected, then there would be no democracy. We should rely on philosophers, such as Plato, on experts and on Nobel Prize recipients. More than once, popes and other spiritual leaders have said that truth is not a matter of electoral majority. Today, the challenges we have to overcome are those related to law-making and those that make freedom possible. We are not talking about some prescriptive rule that is based on decisions made by individuals. And maybe this is the step that will bring us from a prehistorical to an historical state, using a phrase that Marx applied to the proletarian revolution, and a state in which the creation of an *Übermensch* may occur, in reference to Nietzsche. It is important to show that it is possible to deal with all matters of genetic research while at the same time considering a general, worldwide consensus. Here the obvious question arises, how to decide for embryos or for terminally ill patients who are no longer able to decide for themselves, not even if they want to end their lives. This is clearly a set of problems that is very difficult to resolve by clear-cut legislation. Steps have already been taken regarding the issue of euthanasia, for example through the legal provision of a biological will or a declaration regarding what life-sustaining measures should be taken in the case of serious injury. To make this clear, we can apply an analogy with abortion: the life of the foetus is not completely left in the hands of the mother; in order to be able to have an abortion, the mother has to respect certain terms of precaution (no abortion after a certain number of days, and so on) and she must also receive some sort of counselling. It is 'natural', I would say, that the life of the new individual is not just in the hands of the mother or parents.

Reference to Aristotle, and to a non-essentialist notion of 'nature', will be of great assistance in all of these situations. Each one of us has some natural guardians that are both historically and culturally recognized in diverse societies. If someone is mentally ill, the family is informed, and friends and neighbours will be informed as well. I understand that the hostility towards a type of genetic manipulation that does not call for any boundaries for a natural being is motivated by the concern that life could become a consumer object, protected only by the WTO. But instead of relying on an improbable 'natural' rule, would it not be better to consider a positive legislation that does not limit itself to certain traits, but rather falls back on what seems natural or unnatural to an historical community, and that can be formulated after a public discussion and a democratic vote?

To identify the 'naturalness' of birth with pure biological fortuitousness, which can succeed only if we ignore the processes, means that we establish regulations for actions based on what naturally happens; and then, even illnesses, geological catastrophes, any kind of incident, should be respected as the will of nature and, in the end, of God Himself. This fatalistic attitude becomes impossible when science and technology offer us the possibility of changing these events. It is obvious that we need some boundaries, but they must be constructed together, without any illusion of finding them in nature, which would merely be a denial of our individual and collective responsibility.

PART V
Society

Chapter Twelve

On the Responsibility of the Scientist

Dagmar Schipanski

The German Constitution guarantees 'freedom of the arts and sciences, research and teaching' (Article 5, Paragraph 3, Section 1). Science and research are fundamental elements of our free and open society, and in this society no person should have goals or ideas forced upon him. Moreover, our lives are not ruled by 'collective goals', such as those painfully endured for over forty years in former East Germany. In our democracy, we live with diversity of opinion, discussion, and a struggle for consensus. This means that we need as broad a consensus as possible to show us in which direction our society and country should progress.

We need to reach a basic agreement about the foundations and principles that guide our community. This requires an open discussion in which difference and opposition are not suppressed, but are instead solicited, and their ability to solve problems is put to the test.

Society requires first and foremost a firm foundation upon which such discourse may rest. Our core values play a decisive role in establishing this foundation. They are the guidelines and signposts in our lives. They provide us with both a solid basis for behaviour and a means to assess that behaviour. Common values are indispensable for our lives within a community and also help us to cope with new scientific discoveries.

Indeed, today we are confronted repeatedly with changes in our social values. There are many different societal causes for these changes, for example:

- the increase in individual freedom,
- the increase in prosperity,
- the rapid increase and promulgation of scientific discoveries around the world, a phenomenon that is also causing the transformation of the knowledge-based community itself.

In principle, all of these things can be seen as positive. Wrongly understood, however, they can result in the misleading assumption that knowledge and critical thinking are sufficient as a basis for living. Likewise, prosperity and available knowledge are not sufficient for a self-reliant and responsible life, because they require a common point of reference. Nonetheless, everyone must come to terms with these shared values for themselves.

For many, this is extremely difficult. Today, there are many competing lifestyles vying for our attention. Those who break the rules or contravene one of the few remaining taboos are among the ones who garner the most attention. The concept of freedom dissipates into ambiguity, superficiality and blatancy, which accompany us in our daily lives.

This multiplicity causes many to become unsure, lose direction and fall into a crisis of meaning and purpose. Everything appears to be possible and equally valid.

- If, however, everything really is possible, then everything is arbitrary and without inherent meaning.
- And if everything is equally valid, then nothing really matters.

Tolerance is most often brought in as a defence against such a critical and uncompromising view of so-called 'values pluralism'. That defence, however, leaves out one crucial element: tolerance does not mean indifference; rather, it means the conscious sufferance of contrasting convictions.

However, this presumes that a belief is the product of critical reflection. In this way, freedom can fully unfold because it stems from the non-arbitrary. When a society is no longer in the position to determine the boundaries of tolerance and pluralism, then society itself is no longer secure.

A tolerant co-existence of different life philosophies – indeed, one of the signs of our times – does not obviate the need for these fixed core values and standards which form the nucleus of every culture. What is most essential is the foundation upon which these core values are based.

Indeed, the core values that have characterized Europe both politically and culturally over the centuries are rooted in the Christian concept of humanity. At the centre of this ideal is the notion of human dignity. It is the core of our value system and of our make-up as human beings. Human dignity is universal and unconditional, meaning that it is independent of our individual qualities, cultural characteristics and religious convictions. Human dignity is not to be conferred upon humanity by society, and as a Christian I say: God has granted us human dignity. It is His gift to us.

The core values of freedom and equality spring from human dignity. Freedom is the starting point for all ethical, political, societal and also scientific considerations. No person has the right to have another at his or her unconditional disposal. No government has the right to suppress opposing opinions. However, freedom should not be defined as pure individual self-confirmation and self-realization without consideration for others. Above all, freedom means considering the consequences of one's own behaviour for oneself and for others.

Every person is responsible for his or her own freedom in that they are:

- responsible for themselves,
- responsible for their fellow humans,
- responsible for creation.

Freedom and responsibility are thereby two complementary core principles. Not only does our credibility depend upon these principles, meaning how convincingly we justify our liberal attitudes and stand by the foundation of our values, but our entire lives depend upon them. It is not enough simply to postulate human dignity, freedom and responsibility. They must be actively lived, practised and perfected with authenticity and conviction. This is required of every individual and in every aspect of his or her life.

Based on what has already been said, it follows that responsibility is an inherent element of scientific freedom. 'What is once thought can no longer be un-thought', is the essence of *The Physicist* by Friedrich Dürrenmatt. This quote is directly linked to the question of a scientist's responsibility for the results of his or her research, while at the same time it addresses the question of society's responsibility for the social impact of those discoveries.

These questions must be continually addressed with each scientific advance – even in new and currently unknown research directions – and will involve constant and sometimes difficult struggles as scientific advances continue to progress.

As a scientist and engineer, I have often thought about the integration of scientists into society and about our role in the further development of our country, if as Minister of Science I may still consider myself to be a scientist. Moreover, I have thought about these things from the perspective of someone coming from a system in which money was available only for practical research, thereby neglecting basic research and politicizing the humanities. For this reason, scientific freedom is, in my opinion, the most important basic right of our democratic development since 1990.

Now I would like to present the findings of a poll conducted a few years ago by the Institute for Opinion Research in Allensbach. They discovered that 69 per cent of the population believe that scientists provide essential stimuli that will shape our future, and that scientists are the source of our best ideas and concepts. This high esteem underlines the responsibility of the scientist.

To reflect more precisely on the responsibility of a scientist, it is necessary to make some remarks about the character of scientific research. One can technically and soberly formulate it in the following way: the purpose of scientific research is to pursue accurate and reliable knowledge about the world in which we live, to constantly review this knowledge critically, and to make this knowledge accessible to everyone through publication and teaching.

One can also describe it, however, as 'The Wonder of Discovery'. The human spirit is defined by its ability to overcome limitations:

- the limits of preconceived notions,
- the barriers of different languages and cultures,
- the distance between generations and epochs,
- the bounds of current knowledge.

The joy in scientific discovery was expressed by the Greek philosopher Democritus in the following statement: 'I would rather find one single law of causation than be the King of Persia!'

In the past years and decades, the natural sciences have often turned a blind eye to human values. The history of European civilization, however, paints a different picture:

- It was often scientists who, through defiant questioning, undermined the authority that accrued to the powerful, and who – against dependence and domination – cleared new pathways towards freedom. The democratic movement of 1989 was significantly influenced by natural scientists. They took responsibility not only for their own work, but also for society.

- Belief in the totalitarian central plan for business and society stemmed in many ways from the omnipotent fantasies of non-scientists. For most scientists, the fallibility of human knowledge and the limitations of human sciences are part of everyday experience. This knowledge is a reminder to remain humble.

The preoccupation of the scientist to explain the world with the help of theories is driven also by the desire to understand nature. This may sound surprising; only humanity and its works can be 'understood' – and we are only able to accomplish that much because we share our humanity with other humans. But humans – let us not forget – are not only cultural beings, but also part of the universe. Therefore, it is unquestionably appropriate to talk about our ability to 'understand' nature. Through research we experience the natural world as a system of marvellous beauty. Whoever has researched crystals or seen images from an electron microscope is immediately inspired by a feeling of order and beauty.

However, a scientific discovery is in-and-of-itself neither good nor evil. It is new. It is unique. It awaits interpretation and utilization. Every new scientific discovery, as Hubert Markl once said, is 'creative freedom in its own responsibility!' That is an enormous challenge not only for the scientist, but also for the whole society. This responsibility must follow from our value system. Particularly the use and practical implementation of scientific discoveries must be measured by society's basic maxims. The science community is in need of an orientation and identity that reaches beyond economic utility.

However, economic utility should not be seen as inherently flawed. Support for the arts and sciences are made possible by a country's economic strength. In our case, I only need to think about the tight public treasury, which is due to a lack of economic strength.

The responsibility for determining if and how scientific discoveries should be used, and in which direction research should go, lies not only with the individual scientist. An ethical orientation that goes beyond narrow expertise is demanded, because responsibility for the use of research results lies with the entire society. However, particularly with regard to scientific, technical and medical questions, it is often very difficult for laypeople to grasp the facts.

Likewise, scientific and technical developments follow quickly on the heels of one another. In relation to this fact, the former federal president Roman Herzog often quoted Immanuel Kant: 'The need to decide exceeds the ability to understand.' Accordingly, science has the duty to inform society early on about opportunities and risks and to make these transparent. The individual scientist should seek discourse with the general public, not just within the narrow, protected circle of the 'scientific community'.

I am well aware that not all colleagues share this view. I am also aware that it requires a great deal of effort for scientists to present discoveries in language understood by the general public, to witness the 'thumbs up' and 'thumbs down', and to not simply hand over the presentation of their scientific work to amateurs in the media. It requires the work of researchers to take on a new dimension, but this work is urgently needed.

I believe that these efforts are worthwhile. Scientific discoveries no longer take place in ivory towers or in isolation, as in Humboldt's time. Instead, they are developed in collaboration, in discussion and in lively debate. Why should the public be kept from participating in the dynamism of the discussion? Perhaps through such discourse, new and unforeseen questions could arise that stimulate new and unforeseen answers that in turn open the possibility of additional interpretations.

Within this public debate, science should make it clear that both the opportunities and risks posed by new inventions, discoveries, technologies and products will be closely studied and treated in an even-handed way. It should be made clear that the scientific method is dedicated to objective observation. We should never use argumentation that has the tendency to overstate risks and understate opportunities, which is a trend seen in the media.

Overemphasis of risk leads to fear. Fears arise because of the dramatic changes that have emerged in our socio-economic environment and because of the recent increased pace of our lives. As change will be our constant companion in the twenty-first-century, knowledge-based society, we must take these fears seriously. However, fear is a poor adviser for solving the problems of the future.

What is required of such a situation is a serious basis for an open, factual and objective discussion. First of all, scientists and technicians must earn the public's trust. We have to make clear, in word and deed, that not only the laws of nature matter but the basic values of society are important as well. We must clearly state, 'We are not fanatics of progress at any price', but rather that we know, 'Everything that is possible is not inevitably allowed.' We must also make it clear that, as a direct result of recent scientific knowledge and discovery, human life has been decisively influenced, eased, improved and changed.

Of course, today we all use new technologies in our cars and households, and in regard to telecommunications. With a computer, we can retrieve information from anywhere in the world within seconds. Also, think about the developments in space travel, flight engineering and, particularly, in pharmacology and medicine.

Participation in this technological progress is incredibly meaningful especially for the people in the new German states who were separated from technical progress for forty years. We did not voluntarily drive a Trabant for forty long years in order to cultivate a 'special closeness' with rocky East German roads. We like our new cars, good streets, speedy telephone connections and reliable energy.

Unfounded hostility towards technology and science appears to be quite dubious when it is based on ignorance and excess. Therefore, in my opinion, an additional responsibility of scientists lies in informing, explaining and illustrating scientific discoveries in a way that allows them to be used in making policy decisions.

In connection to this last point, I am concerned that science is constantly endangered by politicians who use and ultimately abuse it as a way to secure their own points of view. Politicians in our country have much more to learn about dealing properly with scientific expertise. Scientific discussion is meaningless if one only speaks with those scientists whose political attitudes are known and accepted. Politically formed advisory councils are often treacherous for just this reason. The value of scientific discussion is related directly to the degree to which the scientist has the opportunity to contribute opinions, theories and conclusions that deviate from the views of the client or the enquiring body.

But likewise, it is the right and duty of politicians to make decisions based on careful consideration. Science cannot take this democratic responsibility away from them. Politicians must establish a framework into which our core values are granted legitimacy. Politicians must also, in the interest of the higher public good, set normative limits on research – for example, as expressed in the German Embryo Protection Law. But politics does not have the right to subordinate science to its own purposes.

We all know that many scientific discoveries can be used in conflicting ways. Think about atomic energy: radiation in the correct dosage can be a blessing when put to work fighting cancer. On the other hand, radiation can cause unspeakable harm when used as a weapon. These contrasting effects were not foreseeable at the discovery of atom splitting.

The theme of this conference offers another, similar example, namely human biotechnology. Gene manipulation can heal illness and ease pain. As president of the German Cancer Aid organization, I know how earnestly cancer sufferers are hoping for progress in genetic research. But gene manipulation can also irreversibly and harmfully alter our genetic make-up. For this reason, human biotechnology requires the highest possible sensitivity because by using it humanity appears to be able to alter itself. For the first time in the history of humankind, our creative freedom allows us to alter the human genetic blueprint in a calculated way.

You probably know the prophecy of John Nesbitt, an American researcher, concerning the future: just as the last twenty years have been the Age of Microelectronics, so will the next twenty years be the Age of Biology. Based on my recent work in microelectronics, I must agree.

Thus, it is that much more important that scientific knowledge is made public and discussed in a timely fashion – just as we are doing here. These public discussions must not wait until society is confronted with concrete consequences. For this reason, I find this conference here at the Wartburg so important and essential for the debate in our country. I am particularly pleased that the bishops of our two largest churches, Catholic and Protestant, are taking part.

Research in gene technology and the subsequent processing of its results must always be guided by ethics within the scientific process. Interdisciplinary cooperation is required because discoveries in modern research are produced most often across traditional disciplinary boundaries. In particular, bridging science and the humanities is indisputably necessary. It is crucial that those in the humanities have equal status as dialogue partners when discussing the social and ethical questions of modern science.

The university is the best place for this because it brings together the various disciplines (for example, biology, physics, mathematics, chemistry, theology, psychology and philosophy). In 2002, we founded the interdisciplinary Ethics Centre in Jena. At this point I would like to thank Professor Dr Knoepffler, the director of this institute, for his work.

Beyond interdisciplinarity, bioethical questions have to be posed within an international framework in order to provide workable solutions. The responsibility of scientists does not end at the borders of a country. Science is international and measures its knowledge by an international standard. I should like to clarify this with an example. In August of 2000, the British Ministry of Health published a report that provoked a great deal of discussion. In this report, the responsible minister, following expert advice, allowed the removal of embryonic stem cells in order to help heal diseased tissues or organs. In England, this procedure is allowed up to the fourteenth day after gestation.

As scientists, we have a duty to reflect upon our ideas in a global context. This is a difficult task, particularly since in our affluent society consensus on ethical questions is waning – a situation quite different from that in developing countries. We can sense this clearly in our debates. Here it is particularly important to look across borders. I am, therefore, pleased that we are accompanied by foreign scientists. Sometimes federalism leads us to self-indulgence, and we want to broaden our standpoint with this conference.

The protection of indivisible and inalienable human dignity remains a higher priority than any research or economic interest. Science should, of course, continue to work on methods that do not necessitate the use of human embryos. But these demands should not block all genetic research and the corresponding medical advances. Genetic engineering offers new possibilities to ease suffering and heal disease. Based on my work as president of the German Cancer Aid organization, I consider this a tremendous opportunity.

However, we cannot avoid the most troubling yet most basic questions regarding this type of genetic engineering. How do we deal with advances? Do we reject them on principle and deny their positive aspects? Do we pursue progress without thinking and see it as a goal in and for itself? I consider neither of these two standpoints to be appropriate. The former assumes that there are areas of research that are themselves ethically unjustifiable and, therefore, should never be approached.

We are familiar with such attitudes in the debate about atomic research. They arise not so much from an informed discussion with the subject at hand as much as from the concerns of a culture of despondency and pessimism to which, sadly, we Germans all too often cling. Voltaire once described this propensity to talk things to death with the statement that at the end of every problem sits a German.

The second view highlights a devotion to technology. It favours scientific advancement, but not ethical reflection. The blind faith in progress that can result from this point of view brings enthusiasm and fatalism under the same roof. Einstein's idea that humanity should investigate everything possible is interpreted as though he meant that scientific progress was self-guiding rather than the result of decision-making.

Ladies and gentlemen, on the frontiers of life we arrive at questions that are extremely complex and not at all simple to answer. That also applies to the area of stem cell research. With it, new pathways are open to therapies for currently incurable diseases, but it is the responsibility of scientists to pursue this research for the good of humankind.

Research with adult stem cells or those that have been drawn from the blood of the umbilical cord are ethically unproblematic and extremely promising. In view of their healing potential, we must firmly support this research, as we can accomplish a lot of good with it.

Nevertheless, research with embryonic stem cells presents ethical problems. Following widespread discussion in parliament and in public, with the opinions of the Enquête Commission's 'Law and Ethics in Modern Medicine', the National Ethics Board, the German Research Council, the Central Ethics Commission of the Federal Medical Association, the Church and many others, the German Parliament came to a multi-party consensus.

Parliament had already declared its fundamental opposition to the import and use of embryonic stem cells. It agreed to a compromise, however, in which import was allowed under certain conditions and within a certain time limit. If these conditions are not met, then the question of embryonic stem cell research will again come into play.

We cannot help but continue the debate in order to make decisions based on a more secure foundation. That is why this conference today is so important, not only because we are leading the discussion, but also because we are attempting to present this difficult issue to the public.

Ladies and gentlemen, on what does the future existence of our country depend? We should be conscious that we should attend to, revive and develop this conversation among politicians, scientists and business people. In no way do I want to overemphasize the role of science; rather, I would like it to take its rightful place and hope that the scientific approach, as advocated by Professor Nüsslein-Volhard, gains closer attention.

As scientists, we have a foundation of knowledge provided by the past that heralds an important message. Here I again quote Hubert Markl: 'It is great news that the world orders itself following unifying principles, that there is as it were only one type of world and that the human spirit is capable of recognizing it with a probability that borders on the truth.'

If we acknowledge this, we also have the responsibility to apply it to the well-being of that world. Through this, we are made conscious of the fact that we cannot foresee and plan the future in detail with the help of scientific knowledge. But science can help the future shape itself through creative and independent action towards reasonable goals.

This means neither that can we do everything we wish to do with the help of science, nor that what we can do is something we should strive for – or that we ought to carry out everything that is possible. However, at the same time it means that we share what we have learned, explain it, and gather suggestions for solutions. Natural laws are valid; they should be explored within the context of our capabilities and used to create a better life. Nevertheless, we should be ever conscious of the limits of our own knowledge.

Freedom of research leads us both to the limits of our intellectual abilities and the extent of our influence. This reminds us not only to be humble in dealing with one another, but also urges us to solve the problems we are facing responsibly.

Chapter Thirteen

Society's Responsibility in View of New Possibilities in Human Biology

Ernst-Ludwig Winnacker

In the European Union, a regulation requiring that all genetically modified food be labelled as such went into effect on 19 April 2004. I have always welcomed such labelling regulations because, in the long run, science and technology will only find acceptance if they make their goals and methods public. However, the labelling regulation had little to do with this. The regulation applies not only to products that are made of genetically modified plants, but also to products that no longer contain this genetic material, for example, sugar, starch, lecithin and many others. This means that in the EU there are two kinds of sugar, one kind made from sugar beets and the other from genetically modified sugar beets. The same is true of lecithin, which can be made from normal soybeans or from genetically modified ones. The differences between the two types suggested by the label are not verifiable or explainable because they do not exist. For this reason, the labelling regulation forces itself *ad absurdum*. The only consolation is that the consumers soon ignore the smallprint, just as they learned to ignore labels for chemical additives in our food that were even printed in menus but have long since disappeared. It is unfortunate that the theme of transparency is treated so flippantly, because in the end the damage is done to society's understanding of science and technology. Maybe it is treated this way on purpose because he currently existing draft of the amendment to the Genetic Engineering Law can also justifiably be labelled as a 'preventative law' within the scope of agricultural genetic engineering. However, this is another matter.

Science has at least two other problems to confront, namely the speed of progress and how the risks brought about by the new biotechnological possibilities (Hans Jonas spoke about bio-genetic arts) could impact human beings. The rapid pace of progress in the field of biotechnology and other domains has become commonplace. For example, in the early 1980s, embryonic stem cell lines in mice were derived for the first time. It took seventeen years (1998) for this procedure to succeed in human beings. And recently, human embryos were even derived from cloned embryos. Here is another case. When the suggestion was made to sequence the human genome in the mid-1980s – that is, to read it building block for building block – it would have taken ten thousand years to finish this project with the technology available back then. However, it was completed in 2001, or rather 2003. Meanwhile, genetic data for more than 130 living organisms is now available, among them the genomes for mice and rice.

This accelerated tempo rouses expectations that cannot be met. For example, the sequenced genes carry information about protein components that can be derived from them, but not about their interactions. However, it is worthwhile to be acquainted with these interactions if we want to understand the mechanisms that cause cancer, cell growth, the building of forms in a biological sense or senescence. We can identify these interactions, yet without knowing which pairings should be assigned to which signalling pathway. Analyses of this kind require time because they deal with complex systems and because they often necessitate the development of new technology. The fact that (often self-indulgent) promises made by scientists cannot be kept falls under the heading transparency, which has already been mentioned.

Of course, our actions have an increasing impact on people and lead to a process in which we must consider what we can do, what we would like to do, and what we are permitted to do. Attempts to cross the boundaries at the beginning and end of life are proving to be particularly difficult and captious. In the mid-1990s, a small group of colleagues from the University of Munich and I tried to develop a dialogue, assessment and arbitration model. In this model, the various interventions in humans, including the production and use of genetically modified insulin, particular uses of gene therapy and euthanasia, are measured within basic parameters or tenets such as human dignity, the professional ethics of doctors, the term 'sickness', and the ethics of scientists. To name a few examples: human dignity is called upon because it forbids the instrumentalization of a human being for the interests of others. This means that it puts a patient's dignity above all else, and without his or her permission no intervention or procedure can be carried out. Or: when having to consider between the basic right to human dignity or the freedom of research, human beings always come out ahead. With regard to a doctor's professional ethics, human dignity must also be in the foreground of all medical-related actions. This cannot be questioned either by the increasing demands of the patients or the scientific and financial interests of the doctors. An example from the field of genetic therapy can shed more light on this. In 1999, an adolescent died as the result of an overdose of an adenoviral vector (Somia & Verma 2000: 91–9). The high dose was a type of control experiment and was scientifically but not medically justified. Later, it emerged that the doctors involved were co-owners of the biotechnical company that financed the experiments. Since then, the field of gene therapy has recovered very slowly. In any case, there are currently certain serious failures of the immune system that can only be treated with gene therapy.

I now want to return to our escalation model. It allows us to measure the various types of genetic interventions in humans within the given parameters, and from that we can, to some extent, make a list ranking the weight and depth of these interventions. This model, however, was developed before interventions such as euthanasia and therapeutic cloning were at the centre of the debate. So, the question must be asked whether the model is truly universally applicable. I would now like to test it on the example of euthanasia.

Euthanasia is by no means a new issue. Lately, the euthanasia-friendly laws in Belgium and the Netherlands have reminded us of this. The topic has also been pushed to the foreground because of imminent demographic changes. Studies from the Max Planck Institute (MPI) for Demography in Rostock have made it clear that our life expectancy, contrary to former belief, is not moving towards a maximum, but instead is continually rising (Oeppen & Vaupel 2002: 1029–31). For the last 160 years, it has increased by approximately three months per year, or rather two-and-a-half years every decade. This means that in 2050, the life expectancy for women, which insurance companies and pension funds now set at *c*. 87 years, will increase to *c*. 102 years. Because of this, the number of centenarians in Germany will increase from 11,500 to 130,000 by the year 2050. This is more than a tenfold increase. The indisputable facts make it easier for supporters of active euthanasia to hide their opinions on this matter behind an alleged need to save health care costs. However, there is a relatively low number of 'physician-assisted suicides' according to a US study from 1998. The fact that discussions about these questions are so one-sided has increased pressure on the elderly to see themselves as inferior and mere burdens to society. This is completely outrageous.

Instead, we should try to create conditions that do not even allow the desire for active euthanasia to be expressed. This means organizing and making available appropriate pain therapy and assisted dying in terminal cases. However, we must also take a risk in trying to break the vicious circle between ageing and sickness. For many, this battle seems already lost because of the complex nature of degenerative diseases that indeed represent the risks of old age. However, this fight has just begun.

Just recently, the first signal pathways were found whose failure is responsible for the big killers like breast cancer or colon cancer. Based on these insights, pharmaceuticals such as Gleevec or Herceptin were produced which have revolutionized certain treatments of rare forms of cancer. Therapies using embryonic and adult stem cells are still in the early stages of development, but they remain promising. Nevertheless, I do not believe that cancer will be conquered within twenty years, as claimed by the president of Pfizer. We have heard this all too often, but this does not mean that we cannot see the light at the end of the tunnel. In this way, it is clear that reflections on issues like euthanasia are all too one-sided. Instead, discussions should be conducted as in our dialogue model, in which various principles can be seen in overview; through this, we can find new outlets. A look just at the inviolable principle of human dignity of dying patients can steer the attention all too often onto the economy of the end of life instead of reminding doctors and researchers of their duty. Likewise, one can hide oneself all too well behind the term human dignity.

Let's move now to the debate concerning the beginning of life. The discussion about issues regarding the beginning of life and human dignity flares up continually. For example, in November 2003 the EU Parliament voted to support embryo research without a regulation regarding a cut-off date. Consequently, the danger was and is that projects could be funded with EU money, which, in turn, supports activities and research that are illegal in Germany. However, it gets worse: in late February 2004, scientists in South Korea successfully established an embryonic stem cell line from cloned human embryos. With that, the door has been opened to the possibility of what is called therapeutic cloning, at least from a scientific perspective. I have also heard the term 'research cloning', but this does not make the problem any less complicated. In this case, how profound is the intervention on human beings?

The use of human ova and embryos is a prerequisite for therapeutic cloning. On the one hand, there is the position that maintains that fertilized ova have a right to human dignity, and on the other hand, there are those who argue that an embryo is inviolable only when it is implanted in the mother. These two points of view are clearly irreconcilable. The German Research Foundation (DFG, *Deutsche Forschungsgemeinschaft*) triggered a debate with the suggestion that human embryos could be used for the establishment of human stem cell lines, but only surplus embryos. Consequently, the DFG went down the path of an ethics of deliberation that opposes the arbitrary acknowledgement of an embryo's dignity with an alternative. According to this alternative, embryos should not be produced for research purposes as such, but only those embryos that for whatever reason have not been chosen for implantation will be made available. Both then and now, therapeutic cloning requires a large pool of embryos, which we have seen from the research in South Korea. For this reason, it is not just about the embryo's dignity, but also about the woman's job as a supplier of ova. Women produce a small number of ova during a monthly cycle, which means that in order to produce 10 or 12 ova, a woman must undergo major hormone therapy. A total of 34 women had to undergo this type of hormone treatment in order to carry out the experiment in South Korea. Even though it had nothing to do with fulfilling their wish for a child, they agreed to the terms of the experiment. However, the women also had a 4 per cent risk of becoming infertile, which to some may seem acceptable. We must also consider the following questions. Should hormone therapy be carried out for research purposes alone? Are personal consent and research goals enough to allow a breach of the Hippocratic Oath? Before we as a society can find clear answers to these questions, we must first know what we are getting ourselves into.

For me, a completely different aspect of therapeutic cloning comes to the foreground, namely its precarious scientific background. Therapeutic cloning is more than just nucleus transfer, which both is practicable and therefore can be optimized. It also involves the reprogramming of the genotype of the transferred nucleus. A human being is made up of more than 300 cell types, whose nuclei all contain the same genetic information. However, the information is activated in different ways. For example, because hair should not grow on the liver, the gene for hair growth is switched off in these cells. What is more, in highly specialized cells sometimes all genes that are characteristic in the totipotent embryo phase are turned off. When the nucleus of such a cell comes into contact with an ovum, these 'switched-off' cells must be switched on again. This means that the chemical modification that led to this 'switching-off' must be reversed. Of course, this is easier said than done because of the numerous and serious deformities associated with animal experiments. In this respect, very little has changed in the nine years since Dolly was cloned. One could certainly argue that the standards for cloning an entire animal from an embryo are much higher and should be disparately higher than the standards for creating some embryonic stem cells that are only meant to develop into a certain cell type. However, I am not so sure. In the latter instance, for example, deformities do not play a role. The molecular traces from the reprogramming are already present at this stage and could lead to abnormal growth or apoptosis, a form of programmed cell death. As long as the reprogramming that takes place during nucleus transfer is reminiscent of a stochastic method, experiments on human beings are not justifiable. In this case, there is no need to make an appeal for human dignity. Reference to the responsibility of research scientists, which stems from Article 5, Section 3 of the German Constitution, is enough. On the other hand, however, this reference should not put an end to the search for research alternatives and therapeutic alternatives for degenerative diseases. Nevertheless, nucleus transplantation is an interesting and important tool for understanding the problems of both genetic programming and reprogramming. This can and must be carried out using model organisms because only by using model organisms can the necessary genetic and biochemical experiments be performed. With respect to possible therapeutic alternatives, immunologists tell me that just a few hundred embryonic stem cell lines could cover 80 per cent of immunological diversity, while around 1000 stem cell lines could cover up to 95 per cent. With regard to immunological compatibility, it seems that there are alternatives to the benefits of nucleus transplantation.

The escalation model which I have already described is ultimately an instrument of the ethics of deliberation. It represents a differentiated tool that should not open all sluices of science. On the contrary, it forces us to express ourselves critically with regard to certain aspects of gene therapy or to declare therapeutic cloning an unacceptable therapy, at least according to what we currently know and can achieve. The process of deliberation proves very critical when questions are asked about the beginning of life. Irreconcilable points of view may clash: for example, one side says that the protection of life begins with the creation of the zygote, while the other side says that this does not occur until the embryo has implanted itself in the mother's uterus. Those who maintain the latter position, which is held by many scientists and myself included, do not consider themselves to be 'non-patriots' or 'cannibals', but rather we understand developing life in the same sense as Jesus Christ, who said in the Gospel of John: 'I am the Way, the Truth, and the Life.' We feel secure with this opinion because individuality is a part of being human, but it comes into being only after the point in time at which the possibility for the development of twins has elapsed, and because the embryo cannot develop without a third element besides ovum and sperm, namely the uterus. We could continue arguing over a cut-off regulation that the US president introduced for the first time in this context. The American legal system is evidence of a double standard because the legislators have not created any corresponding legal framework. For this reason, privately funded research is unrestricted. In Germany, cut-off regulation cannot be maintained in the long run and, at the latest, will be abandoned when researchers somewhere in the world succeed in turning therapeutic promises into practically relevant results. We should not reproach German legislators for choosing a step-by-step approach, because according to Bertrand Russell, 'The whole problem with the world is that fools and fanatics are always so certain of themselves, but wiser people so full of doubts.' This is in honour of all who entertain doubts.

Bibliography

Oeppen, J., and **Vaupel, J.W.** (2002) 'Enhanced: Broken Limits to Life Expectancy', *Science*, **296**, 1029–31 [PubMed: 12004104] [DOI: 10.1126/science.1069675]

Somia, N., and **Verma, I.M.** (2000) 'Gene Therapy: Trials and Tribulations', *Natural Review of Genetics*, **1**, 91–9 [DOI: 10.1038/35038533]

Winnacker, E.-L., **Rendtorff, T.**, **Hepp, H.**, **Hofschneider, P.H.**, and **Korff, W.** (1999) *Gentechnik – Eingriffe Am Menschen – Ein Eskalationsmodell zur Ethischen Bewertung*, third revised edn, München: Herbert Utz Verlag

Glossary

Medical and Scientific Terms[1]

Blastocyst: the stage of pre-natal development during which the embryo is a liquid-filled ball. The embryoblast (see *Embryoblast*) is a thick cell mass in the middle and the outer casing of the ball is the trophoblast (see *Trophoblast*).

Chromosome: the intertwined strands of DNA that are found in the nucleus. A human being has a total of 46 chromosomes and each parent contributes 23. Each parent also contributes a chromosome that determines the sex of the offspring, called a gonosome. The other 22 chromosomes, the autosomes, form pairs after both chromosome sets have been united during the fertilization process.

Cloning: the production of an identical copy of a genotype, a part of the genotype or a clone (Greek: 'shoot' or 'child'). This means that genetically identical cells or rather genetically identical organisms are produced. The technical applications of this procedure are typically divided into the following two categories:

(1) *Cloning with therapeutic objectives*: the production of tissue genetically identical to the patient for the purpose of implantation;

(2) *Cloning with reproductive objectives*: the production of a genetically identical organism.

Coding: this describes the process of coding amino acid through three nucleotides of the DNA; that is, triplets. In almost all living things, the same arrangements of nucleotides produce the same amino acids. This is called the 'universality of the genetic code'. The order of the triplets determines the sequence of the amino acids in the polypeptide (see *Polypeptide*).

DNA (*deoxyribonucleic acid*): this is the carrier of genetic information (except for ribosomal *RNA*). DNA is made up of four different building blocks, the nucleotides. These four building blocks are composed of one of four bases that are made up of genetic material. In human beings, DNA has a helical, double-stranded shape in which two bases are opposite each other. Because of its chemical structure only two pairings are possible, and the matching bases are called 'complementary bases'.

Embryo: a stage of pre-natal development normally used to denote the period during organogenesis, which occurs after implantation in the uterus; that is, from around the fourteenth day after fertilization.

Embryoblast: the part of the blastocyst (see *Blastocyst*) that develops into an embryo.

Eugenics: from the Greek *eugenes* meaning 'well born'; this is the philosophy that the hereditary traits of a people can be improved through selective breeding, thereby preventing 'sick' offspring from being born. There is also a difference made between positive eugenics (the optimization of genetic material) and negative eugenics (the elimination of bad genotypes).

Foetus: a stage of ontogeny after the process of organogenesis is complete and with that also the end of the embryonic stage. This occurs somewhere around the twelfth week of pregnancy.

Gene: a segment of either DNA or RNA that is necessary for the development of certain gene products, for example polypeptides or an RNA molecule.

---

1 We would like to thank Markus Peuckert for compiling this glossary.

Gene expression: the biosynthesis of a certain gene product; that is, by means of gene-coded polypeptides.

Gene technology: a branch of the biosciences that is concerned with the processing and analysis of genes and their regulators (proteins that control the gene's activities), including modification and diagnostic procedures.

Gene therapy: a form of therapy still in the experimental phase through which genetic diseases are to be treated through the 'back door' with healthy genes. There are two possibilities: somatic gene therapy, where new therapeutic genes are introduced into the diseased cells of a patient and since the germ cells are not affected, the disease will not be passed on to the next generation; and germ cell therapy, where the germ cells are modified before they develop into a human being. For this reason, the modified gene would be passed on to the next generation.

Genetic fingerprint: the use of DNA to identify an individual. The non-coding segments of DNA that are unique to every individual are used for this purpose, rather than the genes that are very similar to all members of a species.

Genome: all of the genes in an organism.

Germ stage: the stage of ontogeny between fertilization and implantation.

Human biotechnology: from the Latin *humanus*, 'human', and Greek *bios*, 'life'; and Greek *technê*, 'craftsmanship', and Greek *logos*, 'doctrine'. This is a branch of the biosciences with the goal of producing and/or modifying human molecules or cells. For this reason, it is connected to IVF, PGD, gene technology, stem cell research, and so on.

Human Genome Project: this was an international project made up of research groups whose goal was to decode the entire DNA sequence in human beings.

In vitro: fertilization in an artificial environment outside a living organism.

In vivo: fertilization in a living organism.

IVF (in vitro fertilization): the fertilization of an ovum outside the body (literally, 'fertilization in glass').

Morula: a stage of pre-natal development at which the embryo is a cell mass made up of 16–64 cells.

Nidation: the point at which a human embryo implants itself in the lining of the uterus.

Oocyte: a human egg cell or ovum.

Ovarian Overstimulation Syndrome: this develops during hormone therapy, which is necessary for the extraction of ova before IVF and which is accompanied by cystic changes in the ovaries and water storage in tissues in the chest and stomach cavities. This occurs in 0.7 per cent of all women being treated, and it can be fatal, though rarely.

PCR (*polymerase chain reaction*): the technical procedure for producing copies of DNA.

PGD (*pre-implantation genetic diagnosis*): the screening of human embryos produced during an IVF cycle before they are returned to the uterus. In the German-speaking world, PGD is often abbreviated as PID. However, internationally this abbreviation is reserved for pelvic inflammatory disease, and it is imprecise because there is also an optical pre-implantation diagnosis.

Phenotype: a term that refers to the particular appearance of an individual, which is to some extent determined by the genotype.

Placenta: the organ that nourishes the embryo and develops partly out of trophoblasts and partly out of uterine tissues.

Pluripotency: the possibility for a cell to differentiate into many cell types, though it can no longer develop into an entire organism.

PND: pre-natal diagnostic; the general term for all pre-natal examinations of the developing embryo or foetus. There are invasive tests, for example the withdrawal of amniotic fluid (amniocentesis) and, under certain circumstances, genetic testing, in addition to non-invasive tests, such as ultrasound.

Primitive streak: primitive axial organ; an embryo's first sign of an organ.

Pronucleus: nucleus of a sperm or egg prior to fertilization.

Pronucleus stage: the stage before the nuclei of both gametes are united; that is, before the gametes come together.

Protein: spatially arranged polypeptide made up of 100 or more amino acids. Some proteins can be modified after they are created (for example, through the division, folding or integration of another molecule), which means that they are able to perform other functions.

Proteome: this refers to all of the proteins in an individual.

RNA (*ribonucleic acid*): ribonucleic acids, similar to a DNA-constructed carrier of genetic information, which serve to transfer information (messenger RNA) to the ribosomes (the production organelle of polypeptides). Moreover, polypeptides are produced through messenger RNA codes. The individual building blocks (amino acids) are then transferred (via transfer RNA) from matching RNA molecules. Ribosomes also possess genetic information that likewise is made up of RNA (ribosomal RNA).

SCNT (*somatic cell nuclear transfer*): a synonym for a particular cloning method (see *Cloning*). It is the transfer of a nucleus of a differentiated cell – a heart muscle cell, for example – into an ovum from which the nucleus has been removed.

Stem cell: a cell that can be divided almost limitlessly, and whose daughter cells are either new stem cells or differentiated cells after division. Stem cells are categorized in the following way: (1) according to their origin into either embryonic or adult stem cells if during a very early stage of development (see *Totipotency*), *embryonic stem cells* are capable of developing into a clone (this would be a form of embryo-splitting). *Adult stem cells* are found in nearly every organ of a fully developed human being and serve to regenerate organs, such as blood stem cells; (2) according to their ability to differentiate into mono-, pluri- and totipotent stem cells. *Monopotent stem cells* (unipotent stem cells) can be limitlessly divided, but are only able to develop into a certain kind of cell. *Pluripotent stem cells* can develop into many, but not all, cell types, and *totipotent stem cells* (omnipotent stem cells, though omnipotency is usually reserved for God) have the capability of developing into a complete organism.

Totipotency: a cell's ability to potentially develop into a whole organism.

Transplantation: the transfer of cells, organs or tissues into another location in the same organism or into a different organism.

Trisomy 13 (*Patau Syndrome*): a genetic disease in which the 13th chromosome appears three times. Boys who have this disease die before they reach age 5, and up to 10 per cent of girls affected survive to 10. The symptoms are severe cranial deformation and brain damage, heart defects, hexadactyly (the presence of an extra digit on the hand or foot) and microphtalmy (abnormally small eyeballs), to name a few. This occurs in 1 of every 10,000 births.

Trisomy 15: a disease in which the 15th chromosome occurs three times. Carriers are not viable and usually die in the organogenesis phase; that is, between the sixth and eighth weeks.

Trisomy 21 (*Down's syndrome*): a disease in which the 21st chromosome appears three times. Some symptoms are mental retardation and a characteristic outward appearance. However, organ deformities are also common and, in differing severity, leukaemia, heart defects (40% per cent) and deformities in the gastrointestinal tract also occur frequently. Fifty per cent of those affected die before the age of 20, and it occurs in 1 of every 700 births.

Trophoblast: a part of the blastocyst that develops into organs that provides nourishment to the embryo.

Zygote: a name for the fertilized ovum after the merging of the pronuclei and after the first cell division.

Philosophical and Theological Terms

Altruism: in the nineteenth century, Auguste Comte introduced this term into the ethical discussion, and it denotes an ethical doctrine in which we have a moral duty to serve the common good, thereby placing the needs of others above our own. (The opposite doctrine is egoism, in which one pursues one's own self-interest, from the Latin *ego*, 'I'.)

Argument: from the Latin *arguere*; in logic, an argument comprises several statements, or premises. The premises are rationally linked to one another and from them the conclusion follows. When the premises are true and the links between them are valid, then the conclusion must be true.

Autonomy I: a term in Kantian philosophy that is strictly dependent on its Greek roots (*áutos*, 'self'; *nomos*, 'law') and denotes moral self-governance. Because everyone possesses the same common rational faculties, an individual is able to (with sovereignty) establish moral laws according to which he (and all other rational beings) should act. (The opposite of this is heteronomy, from the Greek *heteros*, 'the other', meaning a dependence on the will and influence of others.)

Autonomy II: in modern medical ethics (but in other domains as well), this is a synonym for an individual's right to self-determination.

Bioethics: a discipline in applied ethics that emerged in the early 1970s and addresses moral questions about the responsible handling of living material (particularly human beings). As a synonym for medical ethics, it is understood in the following three ways: (1) as a synonym for medical ethics (as used in this book); (2) as a synonym for utilitarian medical ethics; and (3) as a broader term that includes problems that are usually addressed in ecological ethics.

Conclusion: a term in logic (see also *Argument*).

Conflict/conflict situation (*bioethical*): from the Latin *confligere*, 'to clash' or 'to fight'; in ethics, it refers to situations in which contradictory needs, norms and values clash. One of the most important tasks in ethics is to solve these conflicts. Conflicts then turn into dilemmas (see below) when they cannot be resolved without violating a binding moral principle.

Conscience: according to certain ethical theories, particularly High Scholasticism (Thomas Aquinas), human beings have the fundamental ability to differentiate between right and wrong (conscience as synderesis); that is, an inner 'voice' (Latin, *conscientia*).

Descriptive: the opposite of normative (see below).

Dilemma: situations in which action is incompatible with binding moral principles.

Dualism: within the context of the theory of interactionist substance dualism according to Plato and Descartes, dualism is a position that claims that the body and soul are two independent entities that interact with each other, meaning they can also be related to each other.

End in itself (Selbstzweck): a Kantian term that states that a human being is not just a means, but should always be seen as an end in itself. This means that human beings have a right to the respect of their dignity, which cannot succumb to the interests of commodity.

Entity: from the Latin *entitas*, that which is granted the nature of being; a term in scholastic philosophy that refers to real things (including living things).

Equality, basic: basic equality means that all human beings are equal relative to their basic needs and freedom. However, it does not mean that all people should be treated the same in all situations.

Ethics, philosophical: from the Greek *ethos*, ‘practice’, ‘custom’; this is a philosophical discipline that attempts methodically to answer questions about how we should act and why. For this reason, it is associated with reflections about ethical terms such as ‘good’ and ‘action’. However, there are a number of different approaches. It can also be used as a synonym for moral philosophy.

Extension problem: from the Latin *extendere*; in the case of bioethics, this problem is centred on the question of who has the right to human dignity.

Gradualism: the belief that the various developmental stages at the beginning of life should be morally assessed in different ways. This would then mean that a human embryo would not have the same right to human dignity or enjoy the same moral status as a human being who has already been born.

Hylomorphism: an ontological position that is concerned with the nature of existence. According to this theory, everything that exists is made up of form (from the Greek *morphä*, ‘form’ or ‘shape’) and material (from the Greek *hylo*). What this means is that there can only be already formed material; that is, form and material are two sides of one coin (including living things). Within the mind–body debate, hylomorphism differs from both substance dualism (see *Dualism*) and monism, which reduces all things to one essential substance. In physical monism, everything is reduced to small physical particles.

Imperative: since Kant, this term has been used as a normative moral obligation within the ethical domain. It takes the form of a categorical imperative in which what should be done is turned into an unconditional and objective moral obligation.

Implementation problem: a problem relating to how to socially *enforce* certain rules and norms. It should not be mistaken for the application problem, which deals with the question regarding how these rules and norms can be *put into practice* in concrete situations.

Individual I, conceptual: from the Latin *individuus*, ‘inseparable’ or ‘indivisible’, and Greek *átomos*; this refers to an indivisible substance.

Individual II, scientific: this is used to refer to a living thing that has the ability to develop from within itself or to maintain its stability.

Individual III, philosophical and theological: the portrayal of human beings as individuals is a major achievement of Western philosophy. Human beings are not just members of a kind or species, as in biology; rather, they are aware of their individuality and uniqueness, which results from the distinct way in which they live. According to Augustine, a Church Father and important philosopher in the Christian tradition, personhood represents the support structure needed for individuality. Personhood is founded in the fact that man is called through the Word of God, and he answers Him.

Logical fallacy: an error in logical argument that is independent of the truth of the premises. The most famous kind of logical fallacy is a naturalistic fallacy in which a normative conclusion is drawn from descriptive statements (metaphysical or empirical), and the reason for the normativity is not explained (also called an ‘is–ought fallacy’, as formulated by David Hume). This differs from Moore’s more narrowly defined naturalistic fallacy by which ‘morally good’ is defined using empirical or metaphysical terms, though without mentioning how this is possible.

Metaphysics: a branch of philosophy that addresses philosophical questions that cannot be answered by science; for example, why does anything exist at all? Classically, a difference is made between general metaphysics, which treats existence as such, and specific metaphysics, which deals with questions about humankind (philosophical anthropology), the world (philosophical cosmology) and God (philosophical theology).

Moral: from the Latin *mos*; a material answer to the question regarding how we should act.

Moral Philosophy: a synonym for philosophical ethics; however, it is more precise than the term 'philosophical ethics' because it deals with questions that are terminologically correct meta-ethical questions. For example, what does the term 'good' mean?

Natural Law Theory: a group of philosophical and theological concepts according to which human nature, by virtue of its (God-given) rationality, recognizes a natural moral code from within.

Normative: from the Latin *norma*, 'criteria' or 'rule'; the term for an ethical approach which attempts to establish rules and standards relating to how to live a moral life.

Ontology/ontological: from the Greek *onto*, 'existence', and *logos*, 'rational discourse'; a philosophical discipline that studies 'being' and 'existence'. Ontology according to Aristotle and Thomas Aquinas is a hylomorphistic (see *Hylomorphism*) substance ontology, which assumes that there are both occurrences and substances (see below).

Overlapping consensus: a term from the philosophy of John Rawls, who maintains that an important goal of modern philosophy should be that persons of various religious beliefs and worldviews work together to solve pressing social issues. Furthermore, these solutions should be universally acceptable irrespective of personal conviction.

Person: from the Latin *persona*, 'role', 'mask' and 'personality', though later used to mean 'individual' and 'human being'; a theological and philosophical term, particularly in modern practical philosophy, which characterizes humans as morally capable beings who can be ascribed with word and deed.

Potentiality: from the Latin *posse*, 'to be able to'; a term that is interpreted in a number of different ways: potentiality as a logical possibility, as passive, as active in general, as active in a living organism. This last definition, which is of particular importance in the discussion about the moral status of human embryos and foetuses, is very closely related both to Aristotle's and Thomas Aquinas's understanding of ontology because an organism already has a dispositional potential to become everything that it will eventually be. However, with respect to human embryos and foetuses, Thomas Aquinas would say that they do not yet have an active potentiality; rather, it is passive.

Premise: see *Argument*.

Self-determination/self-governing: see *Autonomy* (*I* and *II*).

Simultaneous ensouling: the belief that a being receives a soul at the moment of fertilization.

Solidarity of Species, for human beings: this is the theory that members of the species *Homo sapiens* should pledge solidarity to each other; or, in other words, they should recognize each other's human dignity.

Soul: a term in philosophy and theology. As a philosophical term and within the context of the mind–body problem, a soul refers to the fact that a human being understands itself to be a living thing that acts consciously. The controversial question is concerned with whether these conscious acts correspond to a separate entity (this is the position of substance dualists; see below) or if the soul is to be understood as part of the body (this is the position of hylomorphists; see *Hylomorphism*). And yet a third camp, made up of the physical monists, believes that the soul is reducible to something physical. In Christian and Muslim theology, it is generally believed that the individual soul lives on after the physical death.

Speciesism: from the Latin *species*; a term introduced by Peter Singer. It indicates that it is immoral to give human beings preferential treatment just because they belong to the species *Homo sapiens*.

Subject: from the Latin *sub*, 'under', and *iectum*, 'thrown'; a philosophical term that is often used to characterize human beings as rational beings, who are capable of moral action.

Substance: from the Latin *sub*, 'under' and *stare*, 'stand'; a term from scholastic ontology (see *Ontology*) anticipated theoretically in Aristotelian philosophy according to which all things have a concrete determinable 'primary matter' (first substance) and take on a 'substantial form' (second substance). Unlike states and characteristics, which can change, the substantial form of things and living beings remains constant. For example, Peter as primary matter (first substance) is recognizable as a human being (second substance). In the course of the history of philosophy, the use of this term has gone through many changes.

Substance dualism: see *Dualism*

Substance ontology: see *Ontology*.

Successive ensouling: the belief that a being does not receive a soul at the moment of fertilization, but rather successively.

Syllogism: see *Argument*.

Theology of mercy: the branch of theology that deals with God's act of salvation towards mankind.

Transcendental philosophy: in this context, it is used as another name for Kant's philosophy, which he called transcendental because its principles do not stem from experiences but rather by transcendence into the knowledge of the world within the subject himself.

Tutiorism: from Latin *tutior*, 'securer'; this is the ethical position that actions should be judged according to how much security can be guaranteed, thereby avoiding damage and loss.

Utilitarianism: Latin *utilis*, 'useful'; a class of ethical approaches based on the maximization of the greatest happiness for the greatest number.

Stages of Pre-natal Development

Time frame	Stage	Description	Size of Embryo or Foetus
0	Fertilization	The sperm pushes itself through the outer casing of the ovum.	
24–30 h	Unification of nuclei > zygote	The nuclei of the two cells merge into one nucleus. From this point on, the embryo is fully protected under the law. The cell also begins to divide.	
3rd day	Development of the morula	It is now a mass of 16 cells called the morula.	
4th day	Development of the blastocyst	Fluid develops in the morula. The cells can now be divided into two groups: the outer layer, which will develop into the placenta and other nourishing organs, i.e. the trophoblasts; and the inner cluster of cells, which is called the blastocyst and which represents the actual embryo, i.e. the embryoblast.	
5th–6th day	Beginning of implantation	The blastocyst moves itself into the mucous membrane of the uterus.	
8th day	Formation of the embryo disc	The embryo flattens out and forms a disc with two rows of cells.	
9th day	Nourishment from the mother's blood	Blood from the vessels of the uterus flows into the area around the embryo (called the lacuna) and begins to nourish the embryo via diffusion.	
10th day	Complete implantation	The embryo is completely embedded under the surface of the uterine mucus, but this has not completely closed in around the embryo.	
12th day	Placental circulation system begins	The blood in the lacuna is regularly renewed.	

Time frame	Stage	Description	Size of Embryo or Foetus
14th day	Development of the primitive streak	The primitive streak, which is a band of cells, becomes visible. This will determine the axis of the body.	
16th day	Development of the blastodermic layer	From the primitive streak, cells push through the two layers already mentioned. Now, three layers can be distinguished: the ectoderm, the mesoderm and the endoderm. These layers will later develop into the various organs, or rather parts of organs. At the same time, the first hints of the chorda are visible, which looks like a channel and will eventually form the spinal column.	
17th day	Neurulation	The chorda induces the formation of the neural plate in the ectoderm. The brain and spinal cord will develop from this neural plate.	
18th day	Initial formation of the brain	The neural plate produces bulges and becomes the neural groove. At the top of the neural plate, these bulges become particularly thick and represent the earliest hints of what will become the brain.	1.5 mm
22nd day	Heart begins beating	The heart tubes, which will later develop into the heart, begin to beat.	
23rd day	Initial formation of eyes and ears	At the top of the neural plate, a channel appears where the eyes will later develop. At the same time, the ear plate takes shape, which represents the earliest form of the inner ear.	
27th day	Initial formation of the extremities	Buds for the arms and legs are now present.	4 mm
51st day	Initial formation of the sex organs	The ovaries and testicles are present, but are not outwardly visible.	

Time frame	Stage	Description	Size of Embryo or Foetus
57th day	Beginning of the foetal stage	All major organs are present. From this point on, the pre-natal process is essentially a maturation process.	30 mm
66th day	Profiling of the face	The face takes on a typical human profile.	55 mm
12th week	Sex determinable	The sex of the embryo is determinable, but only with the help of ultrasound.	
23rd week	In some circumstances, able to survive outside of womb	With intensive medical means, it is possible for a premature infant born at this stage to survive.	
26th week	Able to survive outside of womb	Because of the differentiation of the lungs, premature infants born at this stage have a significantly better survival rate.	
38th week	Birth	Under normal circumstance, the birth takes place at this time.	

Explanatory note:

The scientific–medical terminology relating to pre-natal development is inconsistent. The term 'embryo' (from the Greek *en*, 'therein', and *brýein*, 'to sprout') is usually identified as the time up to the beginning of the third month. At this point, all of the organs are present; that is to say, the process of organogenesis is complete, and nearly all scientists say that at this point the developing embryo enters into the foetus stage ('foetus' is Latin for 'fruit of the womb', 'child', 'offspring'). However, differentiations are made for the period before an embryo implants itself in the uterus. In many cases, the names of the individual developmental phases are used; for example, a fertilized ovum is then called a zygote, which is followed by the blastomeric stage. During this stage, the fertilized ovum divides and on the third day, at which point it is made up of 16 cells, it is then called the morula. However, on the fourth day, the morula is permeated with fluid and is now referred to as an embryoblast. Those who prefer this terminology call it an embryo only when it is implanted in the uterus or when the primitive streak appears.

Indexes

Names

General